Current Topics in Microbiology and Immunology

Ergebnisse der Mikrobiologie und Immunitätsforschung

Volume 40

Edited by

W. Arber, Genève · B. Benacerraf, New York · W. Braun, New Brunswick · L. Brent, Southampton · R. Haas, Freiburg · T. N. Harris, Philadelphia · W. Henle, Philadelphia · P. H. Hofschneider, München · N. K. Jerne, Frankfurt · W. Kikuth, Düsseldorf · P. Koldovsky, Prague · H. Koprowski, Philadelphia · O. Maaløe, Berkeley · E. G. Nauck, Benidorm · R. Rott, Gießen · H.-G. Schweiger, Wilhelmshaven · M. Sela, Rehovoth · L. Syruček, Prague · P. K. Vogt, Denver · E. Wecker, Würzburg

Springer-Verlag New York Inc. 1967

Chronic Infectious Neuropathic Agents (CHINA) and other Slow Virus Infections

Edited by

Jacob A. Brody · Werner Henle · Hilary Koprowski

With 22 Figures

Springer-Verlag New York Inc. 1967

Jacob A. Brody, M.D., Epidemiology Branch, National Institute of Neurological Diseases and Blindness, National Institutes of Health, Bethesda, Md. 20014/USA

Professor Dr. Werner Henle, The Children's Hospital of Philadelphia, 1740 Bainbridge Street, Philadelphia, Pa./USA

Hilary Koprowski, M. D., Director, The Wistar Institute of Anatomy and Biology, Philadelphia, Pa./USA

ISBN-13: 978-3-642-46061-6   e-ISBN-13: 978-3-642-46059-3
DOI: 10.1007/978-3-642-46059-3

Table of Contents

Prelude

HILARY KOPROWSKI

The Wistar Institute of Anatomy and Biology
Philadelphia, Pennsylvania

With 1 Figure

Since only the right word can convey the right meaning, the term "slow viruses" is, in a certain sense, a misnomer. Any infectious process may develop either "slowly" or "rapidly", and its etiologic agents may therefore be arbitrarily classified as "slow" viruses or "quick" viruses. However, what distinguishes more specifically the group of "slow" viruses from other viral agents is not their "slowness" per se, but the ubiquitous, languishing character of the infectious process they initiate in the animal or human organism. The incubation period may last months or years, and the disease itself may progress in a laggardly fashion, characterized by the steady, irreversible deterioration of the host.

Host range for slow viruses may be either extremely broad, including all homoiothermic animals as is the case of rabies virus, or limited to one species of animal, as is the case of Aleutian disease. Kuru primarily affects females of one tribe of inhabitants in New Guinea.

The study of "slow" virus-host cell interaction lags considerably behind that of cytopathic viruses and those causing cell proliferation. The intracellular pathways of cytopathic virus replication have been extensively studied in the immediate past, and the results of these investigations gratified both the curiosity and the vanity of the searchers. The study of the interaction of oncogenic viruses and their host cells, pursued almost as energetically as that of cytopathic viruses, has unveiled many scientific mysteries but has not as yet resulted in the complete clarification and understanding of the process of viral oncogenesis. Cells infected with "slow" viruses are in general neither destroyed nor stimulated to proliferate. For obvious reasons, their functions are impaired but the nature of the dysfunction has as yet not been clarified.

Diseases caused by "slow" viruses are as ancient as rabies (23rd century B. C.) or as modern as Kuru (20th century A. D.).

Because of unusual characteristics of the disease process initiated by slow viruses, because of scanty knowledge concerning the nature of these viruses, and last but

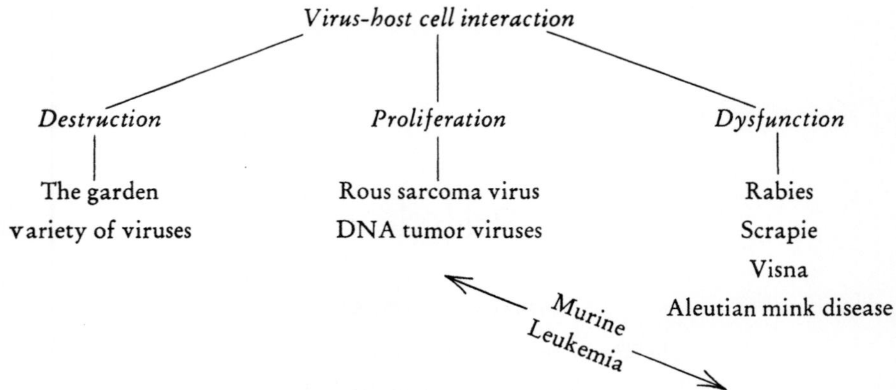

Fig. 1. An oversimplified scheme of virus-host cell relationship

not least, because they are "mod"[1], a symposium on slow virus infections, particularly those which produce a chronic infection of the nervous system (CHINA), was organized on May 4th, 1966 in Los Angeles under the auspices of the American Society for Microbiology. The papers which compose this volume are based on lectures delivered at the symposium.

---

[1] For those who will read this when the slang of the sixties will have been long forgotten "mod" meant "in fashion at the present time".

Chronic Infectious Neuropathic Agents: Possible Mechanisms of Pathogenesis *

RICHARD T. JOHNSON

Cleveland Metropolitan General Hospital and Western Reserve University
School of Medicine, Cleveland, Ohio

In discussing the pathogenesis of disease produced by chronic infectious neuro-pathic agents, three problems are immediately apparent: (1) explaining the long incubation period, (2) explaining the slow evolution of clinical disease and the unusual pathological findings often associated with these diseases, and (3) explaining the role of antibody in the prevention or causation of the disease. In the classic "slow virus infections" of sheep (SIGURDSSON, 1954), visna and scrapie, the incubation period extends from months to years and is followed by a subacute neurological disease lasting for weeks to months. Visna, a demyelinating disease of the central nervous system (CNS), occurs long after the appearance of neutralizing antibody (GUDNADÓTTIR and PÁLSSON, 1966); while scrapie, a non-inflammatory degenerative disease of the CNS, occurs with no evidence of antibody formation (GAJDUSEK et al., 1965). Very little experimental data exist to explain these curious phenomena in visna and scrapie, and discussion of their mechanisms of pathogenesis must rely largely on speculation and by analogy to other diseases. Several viruses, such as rabies, mumps, and lymphocytic choriomeningitis, provide more facile laboratory models and cause diseases in experimental animals which display one or more characteristics of slow virus infections of the CNS. Therefore, studies of these agents may provide some insights into mechanisms of disease production by slow viruses.

Extraneural Phase of Infection

A long incubation period might be explained either by a prolonged period of extraneural growth preceding CNS invasion or by a relatively prompt spread of virus to the CNS followed by a prolonged neural infection before the development of clinical disease. Favoring the latter sequence are the results of experimental studies with scrapie and visna, diseases for which incubation periods of months to years follow intracerebral inoculation. Furthermore, rabies, the classical long incubation period virus, has been found to penetrate into the CNS of animals within 24 to 48 hours after peripheral inoculation (HABEL, 1941), even though signs of disease may

* This work was supported by Research Grant NB-05244 from the National Institute of Neurological Diseases and Blindness, National Institutes of Health Bethseda, Md.

1*

not appear for several weeks. A different mechanism must apply in experimental scrapie in mice in which the agent undergoes a 16 week period of multiplication in the viscera before CNS invasion; nevertheless, many more weeks pass after CNS involvement before disease develops (Eklund et al., 1965). Thus, the extended incubation period appears, in large part, to result from a protracted neural phase of infection rather than from a long transit time to the CNS.

The pathways of virus spread to the CNS vary with different viruses, different hosts, and different routes of inoculation (Johnson, 1965 a). The pathways of spread of the chronic infectious neuropathic agents are probably the same as those of other viruses producing acute CNS disease. Experimental immunofluorescence studies have shown that these viruses may penetrate into the nervous system by neural, olfactory, and hematogenous routes. Following subcutaneous injection, herpes simplex virus in suckling mice invades the CNS along nerves by the centripetal infection of endoneural and perineural cells, a process taking 4 to 5 days (Johnson, 1964). Rabies virus similarly penetrates along nerves in mice, but this spread to the spinal cord occurs in only 24 hours and without the development of antigen in cells of the peripheral nerves (Johnson, 1965b; Yamamoto et al., 1965). There appear, therefore, to be at least two mechanisms of neural spread — one by an ascending infection of peripheral nerve cellular elements and another by a passive movement of virus within the tissue spaces, lymphatics, or axoplasm of the nerve. Spread from the olfactory mucosa to the CNS may also occur by at least two mechanisms: along olfactory nerve fibers leading to infection of the olfactory bulb, or by direct invasion of the meninges via the arachnoid cuffs surrounding the nerves which penetrate the submucosal tissue through the cribriform plate (Brierley and Field, 1948). Immunofluorescence studies with herpes simplex virus following intranasal inoculation in suckling mice suggest that virus spreads to the CNS via both these olfactory pathways (Johnson, 1964).

The hematogenous spread of virus to the CNS is probably more important in most acute virus infections than the other routes. Previously it was thought that a "blood-brain barrier" existed which was impervious to virus particles, but it is now apparent that no discrete anatomical barrier exists. Ferritin macromolecules injected intravenously readily pass through cerebral capillary endothelial cells, traverse the basement membrane and are found within the cytoplasm of glial cells within the CNS (Bondareff, 1964, and it is probable that small virus particles pass through the blood-brain junction in a similar way. Albrecht's immunofluorescence studies of tick-borne encephalitis virus both in mice and chick embryos show that hematogenous spread of virus to brain occurs without evidence of infection of vascular endothelial cells (Albrecht, 1960, 1962). Conversely, infection of endothelium can provide an alternative mechanism for blood-borne infection. Sindbis virus grows initially in vascular endothelial cells, and infection of parenchymal cells of the brain follows the infection of cerebrovascular endothelium (Johnson 1965c). In addition, some viruses may spread indirectly to the CNS from blood via the spinal fluid either by growth in or leakage through the choroid plexus.

The routes of spread of agents leading to chronic or subacute CNS disease are uncertain but, by analogy, neural, olfactory, and hematogenous pathways must be considered. A prolonged incubation period could result from delay along any of the pathways, but present evidence suggests that the long incubation period results primarily from a prolongation of the neural rather than the extraneural phase of infection.

Neural Phase of Infection

In typical acute viral infections of the CNS, the virus, after reaching the CNS, multiplies rapidly and produces prompt onset of encephalitic disease. The histological picture in the CNS is characterized by cell necrosis followed by neuronophagia (phagocytosis) and perivascular and meningeal infiltration of inflammatory cells. These pathologic reactions are presumably the response to neuron lysis.

This classical pathology of viral encephalitis does not develop even in some relatively acute viral infections such as rabies in mice and mumps in hamsters. In both of these experimental systems, fluorescent antibody studies show a rather prolonged period of virus antigen development in infected neurons, and even after the onset of the disease these infected cells remain morphologically intact (JOHNSON and MERCER, 1964; JOHNSON, in prep.). Little or no evidence of cell necrosis or neuronophagia is found, and in the case of fixed rabies virus there may be no perivascular or meningeal inflammatory reaction. These then presumably represent examples of disease resulting from cell dysfunction, since the histologic evidence of cell lysis is absent.

Fixed rabies virus infection in mice provides an example. After intracerebral inoculation, virus antigen develops within infected neurons for about 5 days before the onset of disease. By this time neurons show extensive antigen by fluorescent antibody staining, but pathological abnormalities are minimal — characterized only by a mild eosinophilia of some infected neurons. Electron microscopic examination after the onset of disease shows normal neuron nuclei and intact cell membranes. Neurofibrils and mitochondria appear relatively normal, although displaced by large pools of cytoplasmic virus particles (JOHNSON and MERCER, 1964). This virus-cell relationship may not be fundamentally different from the endosymbiosis of rabies virus in cell culture systems, where infection appears to be perfectly compatible with normal cell morphology and normal cell division (FERNANDES et al., 1965). In cell culture systems, lysis and transformation can be readily detected; but physiologic dysfunction cannot be entirely assessed. *In vivo* greater demands are made on cells, particularly on neurons which must maintain the complex motor and behavioral activities of the animal. The virus-cell relationship that appears to be symbiotic in cell culture may in the intact animal produce disease, particularly in the brain which is the most vulnerable organ because of the great physiologic demands made upon its cellular elements.

In addition to the physiologic demands made upon the neurons, other unique features of neural tissue may be important in disease production by chronic infectious neuropathic agents. The specialized function of different neural cells and the variable susceptibility of different cell populations to infection may be important in the genesis of different clinical diseases. For example, the neurons of the limbic system appear to be more susceptible to rabies virus infection (Johnson, 1965b) and this selective vulnerability probably accounts for the characteristic clinical disease. By analogy, demyelination occurring in visna might be explained by a greater susceptibility of oligodendroglia, since these cells are responsible for the maintenance of the myelin sheaths, which represent their cell membranes. In chronic infection of oligodendroglia even a subtle interference with enzyme systems might ultimately result in demyelination.

Another feature which may explain why the CNS is the target organ in some chronic infections is the apparent lack of regenerative capacity of neural tissue. The agents of scrapie and visna have been demonstrated in many tissues of the body; yet symptoms and pathologic lesions are almost entirely confined to the CNS (Gudnatóttir and Pálsson, 1966; Eklund et al., 1965).

In view of the physiologic demands made upon CNS cells and their lack of regenerative capacity, the question naturally arises how these cells could remain infected for months before pathologic changes appear and symptoms become manifest. The recent work of Mims with congenital lymphocytic choriomeningitis virus infections of mice dramatically demonstrates that neurons can remain infected for the lifetime of the animal without evidence of pathologic abnormality or overt clinical disease (Mims, 1966). It remains to be seen if studies of conditioning or learning in these carrier mice would reveal subtle dysfunctions resulting from the chronic infection.

The Role of Antibody

The role of antibody in acute virus diseases is controversial. In chronic infections its role is even more uncertain. In contrast to the traditional action of antibody in prevention or limitation of infection, studies with lymphocytic choriomeningitis virus suggest that antibody causes disease rather than terminates it (Hotchin, 1962). A similar mechanism was suggested in visna where the virus-antibody reaction may occur on the walls of cells in the CNS, causing the cytopathic effects (Gudnadóttir and Pálsson, 1966). Conversely, the absence of demonstrable antibody in scrapie was postulated as an important factor in its pathogenesis (Gajdusek et al., 1965). However, presence or absence of demonstrable neutralizing antibody need not be considered of importance *per se*. Hypogammaglobulinemic humans recover normally from virus infections; on the other hand, infection can progress unaltered in the presence of neutralizing antibody in such diseases as mumps encephalitis in hamsters (Johnson, in prep.).

Mumps virus can hardly be classified as a typical chronic infectious neuropathic agent, but mumps encephalitis in hamsters produced by Kilham's milk strain (Kilham, 1951) does exhibit several facets of slow virus infection: (1) there is a delay of 10–12 days between infection of CNS cells and clinical disease in newborn hamsters, (2) the CNS cells containing demonstrable virus antigen remain morphologically normal, and (3) infection progresses and disease evolves after the development of neutralizing antibody. The disease in hamsters is characterized pathologically by perivascular infiltrates and vasculitis, sometimes accompanied with vascular necrosis and hemorrhages (OVERMAN et al., 1953). Initially, it was suspected that mumps in newborn hamsters represented a post-infectious disease with antibody evoking the vascular pathology. However, depression of the immune response with antimetabolites and irradiation had no significant effect on the disease or its pathology. Fluorescent antibody staining showed that virus antigen did not develop in and around the blood vessels where the pathologic process occurred but developed within histologically normal neurons. As in rabies virus infections, viral antigen developed slowly in small granules within the cytoplasm of neurons without evidence of cell lysis. Inoculations of newborn hamsters with another strain of mumps led to an indistinguishable vascular disease, less extensive development of antigen within neurons, and no apparent disease. This suggests that disease produced by the Kilham's milk strain (KILHAM, 1951) results not from the pathologic changes in and around vessels but from the dysfunction of morphologically intact infected neurons. Neutralizing antibody appears to play no role in the pathogenesis once initial infection of neurons has occurred.

Similarly, in man, fetal infection with rubella virus has been shown to persist in the presence of maternal antibody during gestation and the neonatal period and then continues to persist in the presence of the child's own antibody. The repeated finding of virus in cerebrospinal fluid is compatible with apparently normal mental and motor development (MICHAELS, 1966). Which cells within the CNS are infected remains unknown. However, cardiac and striated muscle of a child dying with the rubella syndrome showed focal areas of antigen in histologically normal muscle cells (WOODS et al., 1966). Whether such infection ultimately clears, continues asymptomatically, or leads to some dysfunction is unknown.

Summary

Experiments with animals and preliminary findings for several human diseases suggest that (1) virus can infect CNS tissue for prolonged periods of time before the onset of disease, (2) varied clinical syndromes can arise from infection of specific cell populations within the CNS, and (3) infected cells of the CNS may be histologically normal or they may show non-inflammatory degenerative or demyelinative changes which were previously regarded as incompatible with an infectious process.

The mechanisms of pathogenesis of chronic infectious neuropathic agents are largely unknown, but it is proposed that disease results from cell dysfunction rather than cell lysis, and unique properties of neural tissue may render the CNS more vulnerable to disease during systemic infection.

Antibody remains an unknown factor in the pathogenesis of diseases caused by chronic infectious neuropathic agents; its presence or absence may be of primary importance but may also be totally irrelevant to the development of disease.

References

Albrecht, P.: Study of tick-borne encephalitis infection in chick embryos. Acta. virol. **4**, 150 (1960).
— Pathogenesis of experimental infection with tick-borne encephalitis virus. In: Biology of viruses of the tick-borne encephalitis complex (H. Libikova, ed.). Praha: Czechoslovak Academy of Sciences 1962.
Bondareff, W.: Distribution of ferritin in the cerebral cortex of the mouse revealed by electron microscopy. Exp. Neurol. **10**, 377 (1964).
Brierley, J. B., and E. J. Field: The connections of the spinal subarachnoid space with the lymphatic system. J. Anat. (Lond.) **82**, 153 (1948).
Eklund, C. M., R. C. Kennedy, and W. C. Hadlow: In: Slow, latent, and temperate virus infections (D. C. Gajdusek, C. J. Gibbs, and M. Alpers, ed.). U. S. Govt. Print. Office: Nat. Inst. Neurol. Dis. Blind, Mono. No 2. 1965.
Fernandes, M. V., T. J. Wiktor, and H. Koprowski: Endosymbiotic relationship between animal viruses and host cells. A study of rabies virus in tissue culture. J. exp. Med. **120**, 1099 (1965).
Gajdusek, D. C., C. J. Gibbs, and M. Alpers (editors): Slow, latent, and temperate virus infections. U. S. Govt. Print. Office: Nat. Inst. Neurol. Dis. Blind, Mono. No 2, 1965.
Gudnadóttir, M., and P. A. Pálsson: Host-virus interaction in visna infected sheep. J. Immunol. **95**, 1116 (1966).
Habel, K.: Tissue factors in antirabies immunity of experimental animals. Publ. Hlth Rep. (Wash.) **56**, 692 (1941).
Hotchin, J.: The virology of lymphocytic choriomeningitis infection. Virus-induced immune disease. Cold Spr. Harb. Symp. quant. Biol. **27**, 479 (1962).
Johnson, R. T.: The pathogenesis of herpes virus encephalitis. I. Virus pathways to the nervous system of suckling mice demonstrated by fluorescent antibody staining. J. exp. Med. **119**, 343 (1964).
— The incubation period of viral encephalitis. In: Slow, latent, and temperate virus infections (D. C. Gajdusek, C. J. Gibbs and M. Alpers ed.). U. S. Govt. Print. Office: Nat. Inst. Neurol. Dis. Blind, Mono. No. 2, 1965 a.
— Experimental rabies. Studies of cellular vulnerability and pathogenesis using fluorescent antibody staining. J. Neuropath. exp. Neurol. **24**, 662 (1965 b).
— Virus invasion of the central nervous system. A study of Sindbis virus infection in the mouse using fluorescent antibody. Amer. J. Path., **46**, 929 (1965 c).
— Mumps virus encephalitis in hamsters. In preparation.
—, and E. H. Mercer: The development of fixed rabies virus in mouse brain. Aust. J. exp. Biol. med. Sci. **42**, 449 (1964).
Kilham, L.: Mumps virus in human milk and in milk of infected monkey. J. Amer. med. Ass. **146**, 1231 (1951).
Michaels, R. H.: Encephalitis and persistent infection in congenital rubella. J. Pediat. **68**, 842 (1966).
Mims, C. A.: Immunofluorescence study of the carrier state and mechanism of vertical transmission in lymphocytic choriomeningitis virus infection in mice. J. Path. Bact. **91**, 395 (1966).
Overman, J. R., J. H. Peers, and L. Kilham: Pathology of mumps virus meningoencephalitis in mice and hamsters. Arch. Path. **55**, 457 (1953).
Sigurdsson, B.: Rida, a chronic encephalitis of sheep. With general remarks on infections which develop slowly and some of their special characteristics. Brit. vet. J. **110**, 341 (1954).
Woods, W. A., R. T. Johnson, D. D. Hostetler, M. L. Lepow, and F. C. Robbins: Immunofluorescent studies on rubella-infected tissue cultures and human tissues. J. Immunol. **96**, 253 (1966).
Yamamoto, T., S. Otani, and H. Shiraki: A study of the evolution of viral infection in experimental herpes simplex encephalitis and rabies by means of fluorescent antibody. Acta. neuropath. (Berl.) **5**, 288 (1965).

Aleutian Disease
A Slowly Progressive Viral Infection of Mink

Lars Karstad

Division of Zoonoses and Wildlife Diseases
Ontario Veterinary College, Guelph, Canada

With 8 Figures

Aleutian disease (AD) is a slowly progressive infectious disease of mink characterized by diffuse proliferation of plasma cells, hypergammaglobulinemia, and persistent viremia. Fibrinoid vascular lesions, neurologic derangements and Coombs-positive anemia are seen as manifestations of advanced disease. Prominent clinical signs are defective hemostasis, poor appetite, gradual wasting and increased thirst. The most pronounced pathological changes occur in the liver and kidneys. In the liver, these consist of interlobular proliferation of plasma cells, proliferation of bile ducts, and loss of hepatic tissue. The major kidney lesions are perivascular and intertubular infiltrations of plasma cells, degenerative changes of tubular epithelium leading to atrophy, dilatation and hyalin cast formation, and hyalin or fibrinoid glomerular lesions. There is a strong genetic predisposition: mink which are homozygous for the Aleutian gene for coat color experience the disease in a more rapidly progressive form than non-Aleutian types of mink in which the course is more protracted, lasting several months or years.

There is no evidence of direct neurotropism of the AD agent. In this respect, therefore, this virus is not an ideal candidate for discussion in this symposium. Several of its attributes, however, are similar to those of agents whose primary effects are on the central nervous system from a comparative point of view something might be gained by considering together all "slow" viral infections, comparing the morphologic and functional changes which they produce.

The Transmissible Agent of Aleutian Disease

Evidence of infection of AD was first obtained in transmission trials in which mink were inoculated with suspensions of diseased tissues (Henson et al., 1962a; Karstad and Pridham, 1962; Russell, 1962). Subsequently, it was found that the causative agent was filterable, passing membrane filters as small as 50 mμ (Karstad and Pridham, 1962; Gray, 1964; Henson et al., 1963) and deposited by centrifugation at 95,000 g (HENSON et al., 1963). It was shown to be partially resistant to formalin inactivation (HENSON et al., 1962a; KARSTAD et al., 1963) and to inactivation by heat, remaining infective in tissue suspensions at 80° C for 30 minutes, and for three minutes at 99.5° C (GRAY, 1964). Recently, mink inoculated with DNA extracted from diseased spleens have developed typical lesions and AD, while controls inoculated with enzyme-digested DNA remained normal (BASRUR and KARSTAD, 1966).

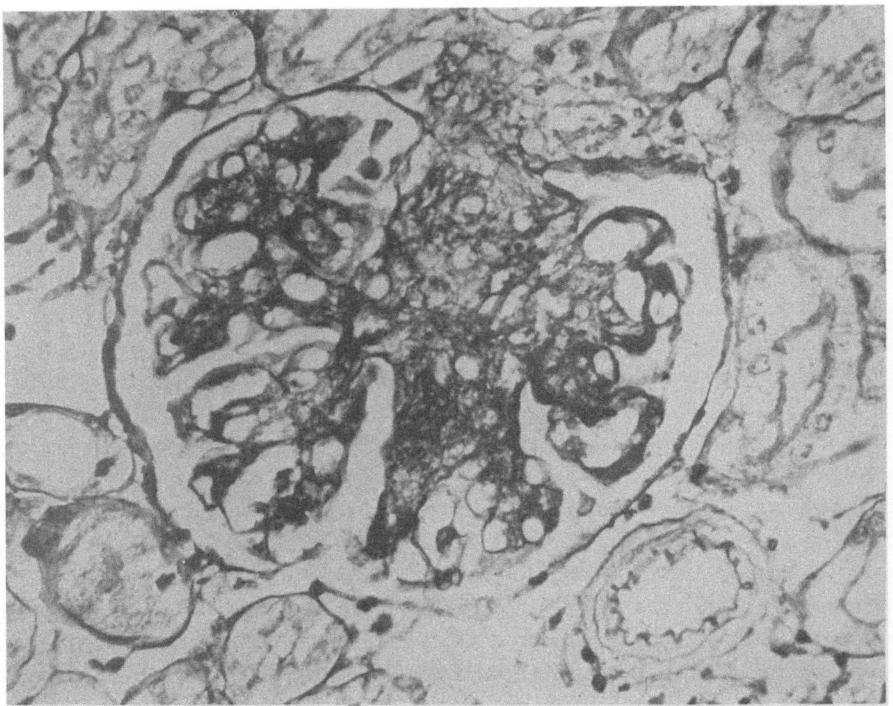

Fig. 1. Kidney from a standard dark mink with Aleutian disease, killed 118 days after inoculation with a diseased tissue suspension. There are marked proliferative changes in stalk and mesangial portions of the glomerulus and thickening of capillary basement membranes. PAS stain. × 750

Mink are the only proven hosts for this virus. Early attempts to propagate the virus in primary cultures of mink tissues appeared to be successful (BASRUR et al., 1963), although these findings have not subsequently been confirmed. The suggested susceptibility of man to infection with the AD virus also lacks confirmation (CHAPMAN and JIMENEZ, 1963).

Transmission of the AD agent among mink occurs both horizontally and vertically. HENSON et al. (1962b), PORTER and LARSEN (1964) and PADGETT and DICKINSON (1965) have published supporting evidence for this view. In our own work, kits born to dams experimentally inoculated with infective materials during gestation have developed AD in early life. In another experiment, infection was shown to spread readily from inoculated to contact mink within the same cage. Thus, AD is not only an infectious disease, it is contagious.

Studies on the Pathogenesis of Aleutian Disease

The pathologic changes seen in mink with AD were described by HELMBOLDT and JUNGHERR (1958) and OBEL (1959). LEADER et al. (1963b) have described in detail the pathologic changes seen in livers and kidneys, the organs most severely affected. A further contribution to knowledge of the pathology of this disease in mink, especially with reference to amyloid and para-amyloid lesions, was made by TRAUTWEIN (1964).

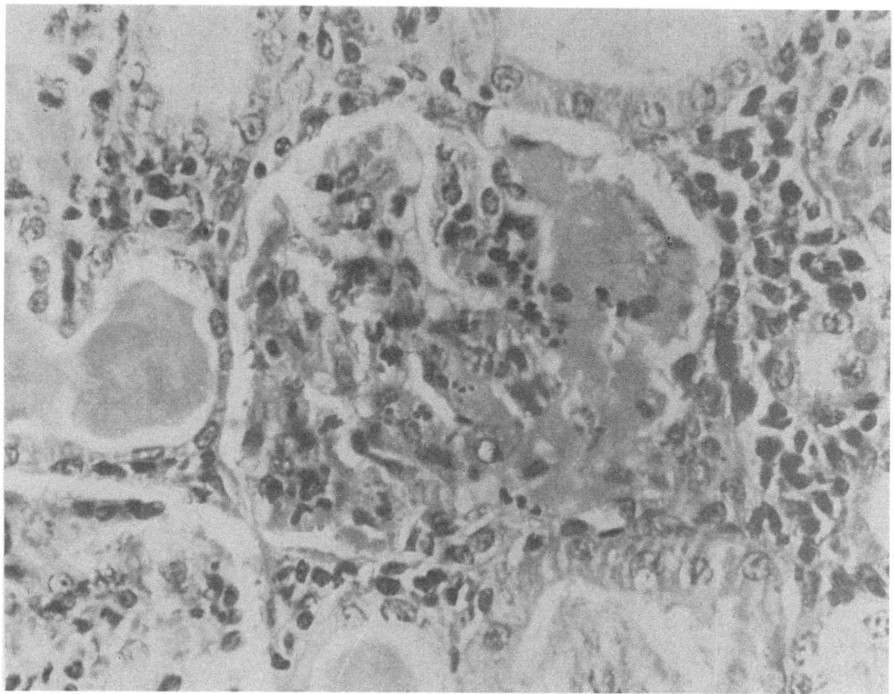

Fig. 2. Kidney from a standard dark mink with Aleutian disease, killed 118 days after inoculation with a suspension of diseased tissues. There is evidence of recent fibrin thrombosis of one segment of the glomerulus, resulting in an acidophilic hyaline mass containing nuclear remnants. Periglomerular tissues contain numerous plasma cells and tubules with hyaline casts. H and E stain. x 750

Sequential studies of the histologic alterations in experimental AD revealed plasmacytosis at an abnormally increased level, first appearing in the normal sites of plasma cell proliferation, the lymph nodes, bone marrow and spleen. Next the liver becomes affected, with proliferation of plasma cells in portal areas, followed by perivascular plasma cell proliferation in renal tissues. In severely diseased mink, perivascular plasma cell infiltrates may be found in any tissue or organ.

Abnormal elevation of serum gamma globulin parallels the plasmacytosis (HENSON et al., 1961; KENYON and HELMBOLDT, 1964). The specificity of this gamma globulin is not known; it may or may not be antibody, or it may contain a variety of antibodies. This gamma globulin does not suppress the infectivity of the virus, since serum from animals with pronounced hypergammaglobulinemia remains infective for other mink (Gorham et al., 1965). That the elevated gamma globulin is not merely the result of nonspecific stimulation of antibody-producing cells is attested by the observations of Porter et al. (1964), who measured the production of antibodies to hemocyanin and bovine globulin in mink immunized

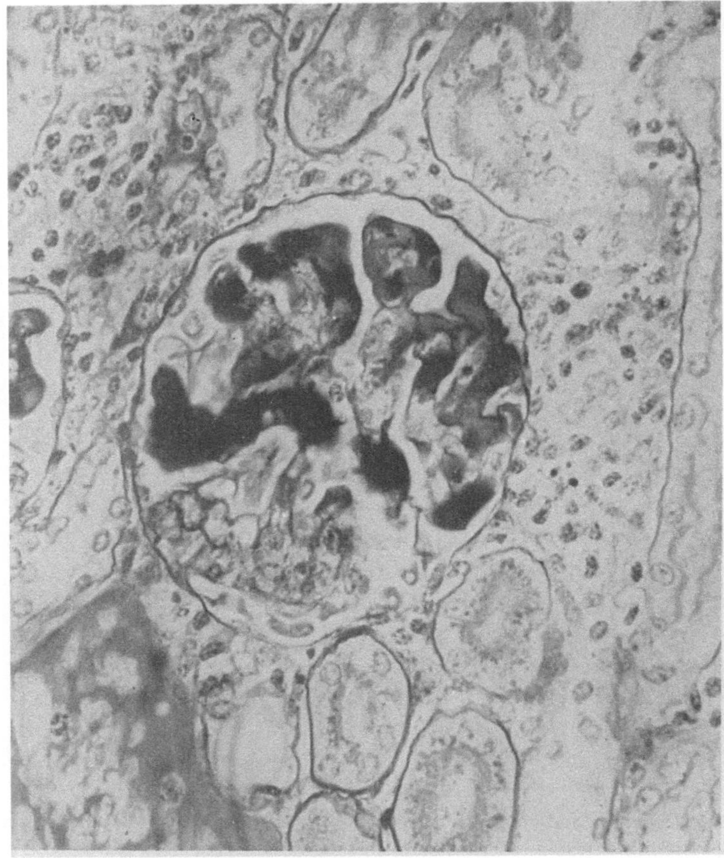

Fig. 3. Kidney of an Aleutian mink killed 118 days after inoculation with a suspension of tissues from mink with plasmacytosis. Fibrin thrombi are present within glomerular capillaries. PAS stain. × 750

before they were affected with AD. Antibodies resulting from such pre-immunization fell rather than rose during development of the hypergammaglobulinemia.

Hyalin glomerular lesions are a constant finding in severely diseased mink (Leader et al., 1963b). These appear to be of at least two distinct types and to develop in different ways:

(A) Slowly developing, periodic acid Schiff (PAS)-positive thickenings of the stalk and mesangial portions of the glomerulus (Fig. 1).

(B) Rapidly formed deposits within glomerular capillaries, staining first as fibrin, later losing their capacity to stain as fibrin and persisting as smooth, dense, nodular PAS-positive masses (Fig. 2 and 3).

The hyalin PAS-positive material deposited in glomerular lesions has not been identified. Resemblance of this material to that found in certain other glomerular lesions, both naturally occurring and experimental, suggests an immunologic basis for its origin (LEADER, 1964; THOMPSON and ALIFERIS, 1964). It is therefore surprising that PORTER et al. (1964) were not able to demonstrate more than trace amounts of gamma globulin and fibrin in affected glomeruli. It is possible that

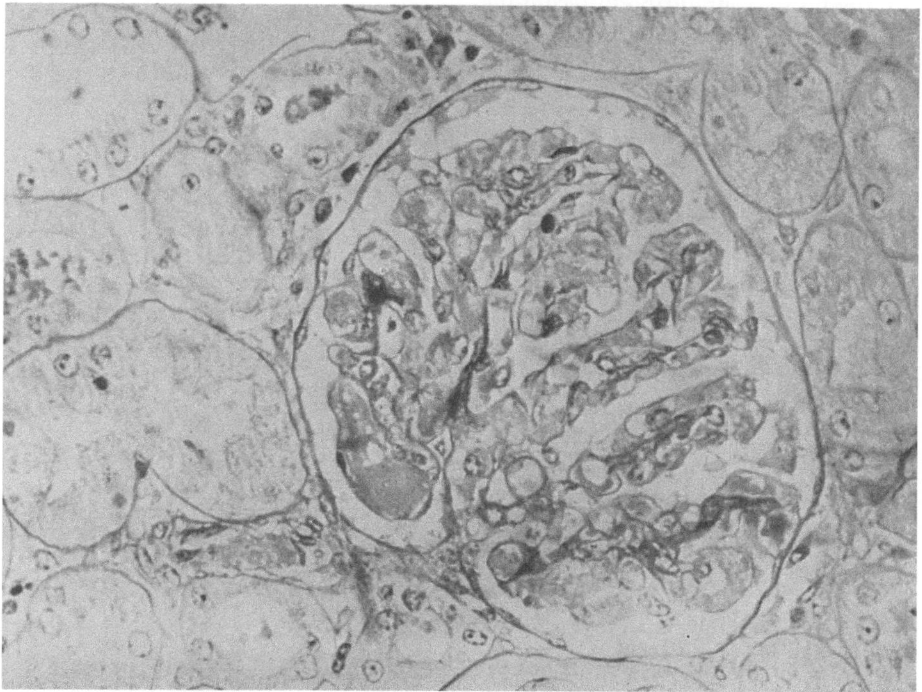

Fig. 4. Kidney of a pastel mink which died 24 hours after endotoxin injection and 35 days after inoculation with a suspension of tissues from mink with plasmacytosis. There are fibrin thrombi within the lumens of glomerular capillaries and tubular epithelial cells are necrotic. PAS stain. x 750

their animals did not have the severe hyalin lesions seen by others in typical cases of advanced AD (KARSTAD, 1965; LEADER, 1964). They noted only the mesangial lesions described as type A, above. It seems that further study is warranted, employing immunofluorescence to look for localization of fibrin and gamma globulin at varying stages of development in the glomerular lesions of AD.

Recent findings on blood coagulation in mink with AD may be used to explain the pathogenesis of the type B glomerular lesions, described above. PHILLIPS and HENSON (1966) report gradual progressive thrombocytopenia in mink with AD. This, together with assay results of other coagulation factors, has prompted them to postulate a process of prolonged intravascular fibrin formation. This hypothesis agrees with the histologic observations we have made. Occasionally we find evidence of recent extensive glomerular thrombosis and AD. More often only a few glomeruli are found which have their capillaries plugged with material

staining as fibrin with phosphotungstic acid-hematoxylin (PTAH) or with Wei-
gert's fibrin stain. Other glomeruli in the same section will have similar nodular
hyalin masses which do not have the staining qualities of fibrin. These are obviously the residual lesions of capillary thrombosis. Aging of fibrin with loss of
typical staining qualities has been described by others (LENDRUM, 1963). Perhaps
these older lesions also lose their immunospecificity for staining with antifibrinogen
by the fluorescent antibody technique.

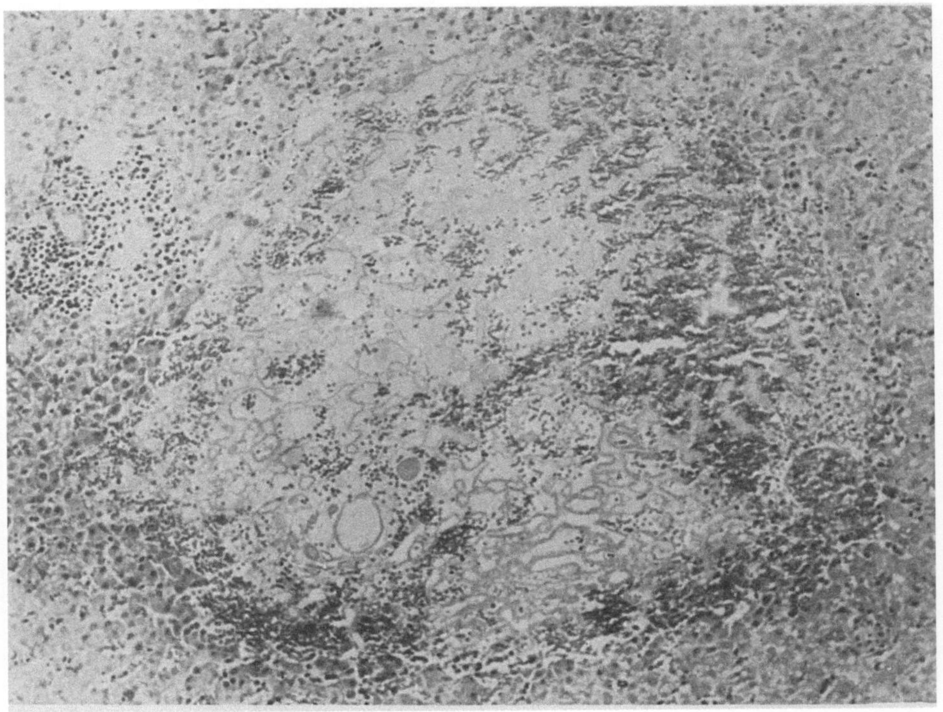

Fig. 5. Liver of the same animal as figure 3. One lobule has been lost through thrombosis and
necrosis. The upper left of the figure contains a portal triad infiltrated with plasma cells. The
central vein can be seen the lower right of the necrotic area. H and E stain. x 190

To gain a better understanding of the role of intravascular coagulation in the
pathogenesis of AD, we attempted to produce the generalized Shwartzman reaction. We found that mink with AD were extremely sensitive to a single injection of *Escherichia coli* endotoxin. As little as 0.2 mg of endotoxin administered
intracardially caused immediate signs of gastrointestinal irritability and pro-
found depression. Mink which died, or which were killed 24 hours after endotoxin injection, were found to have necrosis of germinal centers in the spleen and
lymph nodes, focal liver necrosis, fibrin thrombi in glomerular capillaries, and
patchy necrosis of renal tubules (Fig. 4). Obviously the mink with AD, in developing the generalized Shwartzman reaction, responded as if they had previously been sensitized by a dose of endotoxin or an injection of some substance
which caused blockade of the reticulo-endothelial system (RES).

We may postulate that prolonged low-level intravascular coagulation results in a state of RES overload or blockade. Such mink are then highly susceptible to tissue injury resulting from further intravascular fibrin formation. In support of this hypothesis, we frequently find histologic evidence in AD of extensive PAS-positive and iron-containing deposits within cells of the RES, focal necrosis of liver tissue (Fig. 5) and fibrinoid glomerular lesions referred to as type B, above (Fig. 2 and 3).

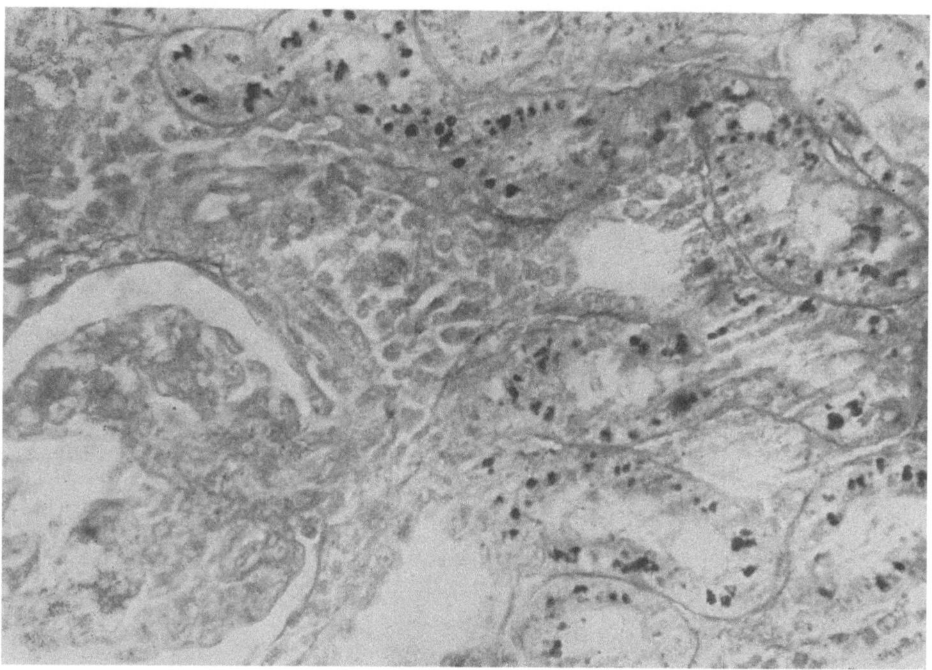

Fig. 6. Kidney of an Aleutian mink killed 97 days after inoculation with blood from a mink with plasmacytosis. Dense granular deposits in tubular epithelial cells contain iron. Prussian blue reaction. x 750

PORTER and his associates (1964) have employed a variety of methods to look for evidence of the suggested autoimmunologic basis of AD. Tests for rheumatoid factor, for lupus erythematosus (LE) cells, and for autoantigens or autoantibodies, using the techniques of agar gel precipitation and complement fixation, were consistently negative.

Recently RUTH SAISON, of our laboratories, found that erythrocytes of mink with AD consistently become sensitized with serum globulins, as detected by agglutination with antiglobulin in the direct Coombs test (SAISON et al., 1966). It is not known whether the globulin coating the red cells is autoantibody, or antibody to some antigen adsorbed to the cell membrane. Positive Coombs test reactions are obtained in both naturally-occurring and experimentally-induced AD, and even in animals exposed by contact only, never having been inoculated with tissue suspensions.

Anemia is a consistent finding in mink in the late stages of AD. This is partly explainable on the basis of the observed uremia and defective hemostasis (Karstad and Pridham, 1962; Thompson and Aliferis, 1964; Gershbein and Spencer, 1964). Black "tarry" droppings are a common finding. Loss of blood by hemorrhage appears to be intermittent or inconstant, however, and not sufficient to explain the anemia. It now seems probable that we are dealing with a hemolytic anemia, perhaps of autoimmune type. The anemia of AD is characterized by increased sedimentation rate, decreased hematocrit and erythrocyte

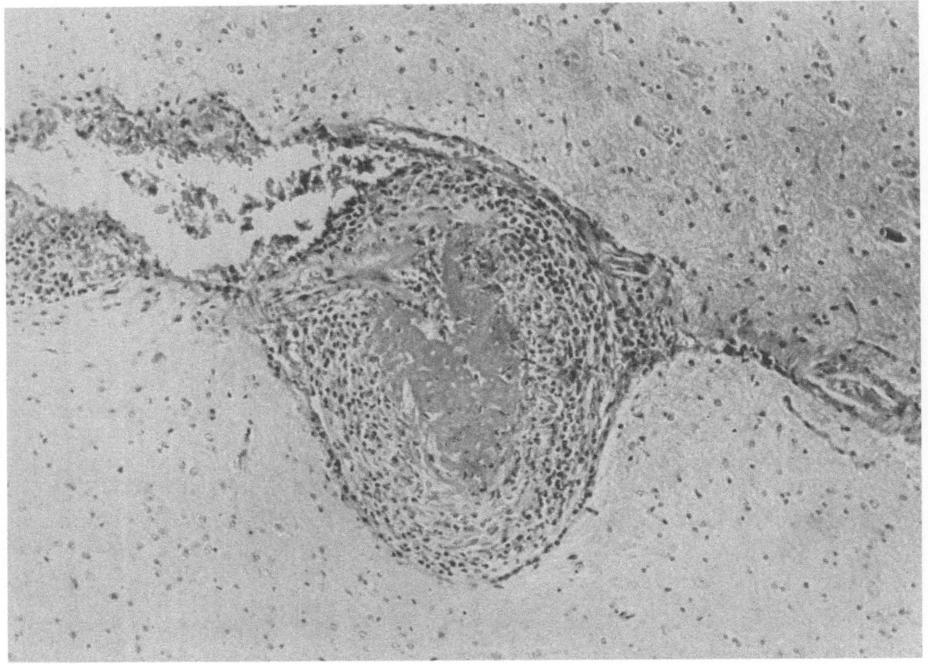

Fig. 7. Cerebrum of mink with Aleutian disease showing nodular fibrinoid arteritis associated with hemorrhage. H and E stain. x 190

counts, and increased deposition of iron in tissues. This iron is found both within cells of the RES and in cells of the proximal convoluted tubules (Fig. 6).

Many mink with severe AD have arterial lesions resembling polyarteritis nodosa (Leader et al., 1963 b; Trautwein, 1964; Karstad, 1965). By immunofluorescent techniques, Porter et al. (1965) were able to demonstrate the localization of gamma globulin within the damaged arterial walls. The mechanism of injury is unknown. These lesions are similar to those of polyarteritis nodosa in man, except that in the AD lesions the inflammatory cells are usually mononuclear leukocytes, whereas in man, polymorphonuclear leukocytes are more common.

The functional and morphologic signs of disease of the central nervous system in AD, seem to be directly referable to vascular lesions. Signs of derangement are variable, depending upon the location of the arterial lesions in the brain.

Diseased arteries have been found associated with perivascular or paravascular hemorrhages, areas of softening, the presence of glial phagocytes loaded with cellular and plasmatic debris, and glial scarring (Fig. 7). Other lesions commonly seen in AD are mild meningitis, perivascular cuffing with lymphocytes and plasma cells, and plasma cell infiltration of the choroid plexus (HELMBOLDT and JUNGHERR, 1958; TRAUTWEIN, 1964). Ordinarily, these latter lesions alone are not associated with clinical signs.

One of the most interesting aspects of AD is the genetic predisposition shown by mink homozygous for the Aleutian gene for coat color. It is now recognized that these animals have an inherited anomaly of granules in granule producing cells throughout the body (LEADER et al., 1963b; LUTZNER et al., 1965). This anomaly was recognized previously in man, and bears the designation Chediak-Higashi Syndrome. Affected animals and humans have defective pigmentation and unusual susceptibility to bacterial infections (LEADER, 1964). Increased susceptibility to viral infections, other than AD, has not been noted. Lysosomes have been identified among the abnormal granules demonstrable by electron microscopy (LUTZNER et al., 1965). It has been postulated that affected cells are unable to digest phagocytosed bacteria (LEADER, 1964).

Discussion and Conclusions

Interesting facets in AD and shared by several other slowly progressive viral infections are:

(1) persistent (tolerant) infection, often with persistent viremia,
(2) coincidence of virus and antibody,
(3) "failure" of immunity,
(4) genetic predisposition,
(5) vertical transmission and familial occurrence,
(6) autoimmune phenomena,
(7) slow inevitable development of disease.

How do these factors act in concert to produce the variety of pathologic alterations seen in AD? A postulated double cycle of pathogenetic events is presented in Fig. 8. The primary cycle of viral infection-plasmacytosis-viral antibody production may be unusual only in its prolonged action. If antibody to the virus is produced, it is not successful in suppressing the infection. Similar "peaceful co-existence" of virus and antibody occurs in visna and in avian leukosis (THORMAR, 1963; RUBIN et al., 1962).

The RES functions to remove antigen-antibody complexes from circulation (LEE, 1964). WEISSMAN (1965) lists endocytosis (phagocytosis), antigen-antibody reactions, virus infections, and endotoxin among the agents which cause labilization of lysosomes within living cells, presumably in this way facilitating release of enzymes into the cytoplasm. Enzyme digestion or partial digestion of native cytoplasmic proteins may create auto-antigens, which are stimuli to further plasma cell proliferation and gamma globulin production. Auto-antigens produced under these circumstances would be of a variety of types; similarly their corresponding auto-antibodies would be a diverse population. Perhaps the damaged lysosome membranes also become auto-antigenic. WEISSMAN (1965) has mentioned a structural similarity which exists between lysosome membranes and red cell membranes. It should therefore be no surprise that antibody to lysosome membranes may cross-react with normal antigens on the erythrocyte surface. QUIE and HIRSCH (1964) have demonstrated hemolytic effects of antibodies to leukocyte lysosomes and the converse, cytotoxicity for leukocytes of

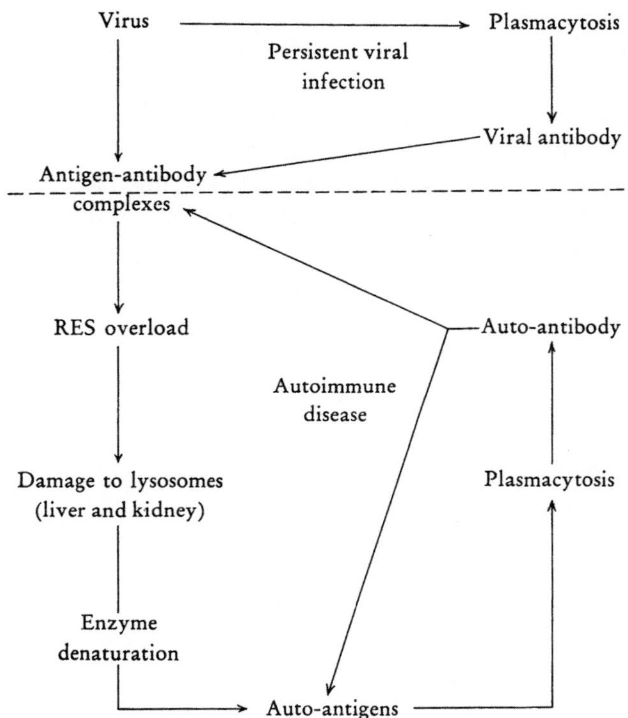

Fig. 8. Schematic representation of a postulated sequence of events in the pathogenesis of Aleutian disease

antibody to erythrocytes. It seems possible, therefore, that antibody to enzyme-denatured cytoplasmic constituents may be responsible for the positive Coombs tests which we observe in AD.

One may pose the question, how does intravascular fibrin formation fit into our schematic presentation of AD pathogenesis? It has been shown that normal RES function is essential for the clearance of circulating fibrin. It is known that intravenous administration of soluble antigen-antibody complexes can cause RES blockade. Furthermore, RES blockade can be caused by an infusion of antigen into a previously hyperimmunized animal (LEE, 1964). Regardless of the agent causing RES blockade, the injurious factor (as seen in the generalized Shwartzman reaction) is fibrin deposition on and within cells of the RES (PROSE et al., 1965). Degraded fibrin is taken up also by endothelial cells of the glomerulus (SIMON and CHATELA-NAT, 1963). Hemolysis and antigen-antibody complexes can contribute to intravascular fibrin formation (LEE, 1964; QUICK, 1957).

We may postulate, therefore, that blockade of the RES occurs in mink with AD (as evidenced by their hypersensitivity to endotoxin), that fibrin clearance is impeded, and that several of the major pathologic changes in AD are the direct result of intravascular coagulation.

Support for the postulated role of lysosomes and lysosome enzymes in the pathogenesis of AD may be found when we acquire a better understanding of the exact nature of the lysosome defect in Aleutian type mink. What is it that makes them more susceptible to AD? Is it cellular inability to digest and dispose of phagocytosed antigen-antibody complexes and fibrin?

BARLOW and HOTCHIN (1963) have reported increased susceptibility to endotoxin in mice with lymphocytic choriomeningitis (LCM). Furthermore, HOTCHIN et al. (1963) describe the development of a "late disease" in LCM tolerant mice; this appears to have similarities to AD with respect to renal lesions and evidence of autoimmunity.

BURNET (1965) has postulated the development of autoimmune damage to the central nervous system in kuru, through viral release of cerebellar antigens during persistent tolerant infection.

We are hopeful that comparative studies on the pathogenesis of the "slow" viral infections will continue to provide useful guidelines for further investigations, leading eventually to complete understanding.

Summary

Aleutian disease (AD) is described as a slowly-progressive viral infection of mink causing extensive plasmacytosis, hypergammaglobulinemia, and lesions typical of an "autoimmune disease". Hypersensitivity to endotoxin is indicative of damage to the reticulo-endothelial system (RES). This, in mink with AD, appears to be responsible for failure of circulation fibrin clearance and intravascular thrombosis. Intravascular coagulation is believed directly responsible for some of the major pathologic changes in AD, such as focal liver necrosis and hyalin glomerular lesions. Coombs-positive anemia develops as a late manifestation of disease. Hemolysis, antigen-antibody complexes, and thrombocytopenia probably all contribute to increased intravascular fibrin formation. It is postulated that excessive phagocytosis of fibrin and antigen-antibody complexes by cells of the RES may predispose to a sequence of intracytoplasmic release of lysosome enzymes, denaturation of native proteins and the creation of auto-antigens. Aleutian disease may represent, therefore, a virus-induced autoimmune process.

References

BARLOW, J. L., and J. HOTCHIN: Hyper-reactivity to endotoxin in mice infected with lymphocytic choriomeningitis. Fed. Proc. 22, (2) Pt. 1, 628 (1963).

BASRUR, P. K., D. P. GRAY, and L. KARSTAD: Aleutian disease (plasmacytosis) of mink. III. Propagation of the virus in mink tissue cultures. Canad. J. comp. med. 27, 301—306 (1963).

Basrur, P. K., and L. Karstad: Studies on viral plasmacytosis (Aleutian disease) of mink. VII. Infection of mink with DNA prepared from diseased spleens. Canad. J. comp. Med. (In press, 1966.)

Burnet, F. M.: Appendix to The changing face of kuru by J. P. Mathews. Lancet 1965 I, 1141—1142.

Chapman, I., and F. A. Jimenez: Aleutian-mink disease in man. New Engl. J. Med. 269, 1171—1174 (1963).

Gershbein, L. L., and Kathryn L. Spencer: Clinical chemical studies in Aleutian disease of mink. Canad. J. comp. med. 28, 8—12 (1964).

Gorham, J. R., R. W. Leader, and J. B. Henson: Neutralizing ability of hypergamma-globulinemic serum on Aleutian disease virus of mink (Abstract). Fed. Proc. 22, (Pt. 1), 265 (1965).

Gray, D. P.: Studies on the etiology of plasmacytosis of mink, p. 65. MVSc. thesis. University of Toronto, 1964.

Helmboldt, C. F., and E. L. Jungherr: The pathology of Aleutian disease in mink. Amer. J. vet. Res. 19, 212—222 (1958).

Henson, J. B., R. W. Leader and J. R. Gorham: Hypergammaglobulinemia in mink. Proc. Soc. exp. Biol. (N. Y.) 107, 919—920 (1961).

—, J. R. Gorham, R. W. Leader, and B. M. Wagner: Experimental hypergammaglob-ulinemia in mink. J. exp. Med. 116, 357—364 (1962 a).

— — — A field test for Aleutian disease. (Preliminary report.) Nat. Fur News 34, 8, 9, 23, 25 and 26 (1962b).

— — — Hypergammaglobulinemia in mink initiated by a cell-free filtrate. Nature (Lond.) 197, 207 (1963).

Hotchin, J., Lois M. Benson, and Doris N. Collins: Late-onset kidney disease of mice with persistent tolerant infection with lymphocytic choriomeningitis. Fed. Proc. 22, (2) Pt. 1, 441 (1963).

Karstad, L.: Viral plasmacytosis (Aleutian disease) in mink. V. The occurrence of hyalin glomerular lesions and fibrinoid arteritis in experimental infections. Canad. J. comp. Med. 29, 66—74 (1965).

—, and T. J. Pridham: Aleutian disease of mink. I. Evidence of its viral etiology. Canad. J. comp. Med. 26, 97—102 (1962).

— —, and D. P. Gray: Aleutian disease (plasmacytosis) of mink. II. Responses of mink to formalin-treated diseased tissues and to subsequent challenge with virulent inoc-ulum. Canad. J. comp. Med. 27, 124—128 (1963).

Kenyon, A. J., and C. F. Helmboldt: Solubility and electrophoretic characterizations of globulins from mink with Aleutian disease. Amer. J. vet. Res. 25, 1535—1541 (1964).

Leader, R. W.: Lower animals, spontaneous disease, and man. Arch. Path. 78, 390—404 (1964).

— G. A. Padgett, and J. R. Gorham: Studies of abnormal leukocyte bodies in the mink. Blood 22, 477—484 (1963 a).

— B. M. Wagner, J. B. Henson, and J. R. Gorham: Structural and histochemical obser-vations of liver and kidney in Aleutian disease in mink. Amer. J. Path. 43, 33—53 (1963 b).

Lee, L.: Mechanisms involved in the production of the generalized Shwartzman reaction. In: Bacterial Endotoxins: Proceedings of a symposium, p. 648—657. Rutgers Uni-versity. Rahway, N. J.: Quinn & Boden Co. 1964.

Lendrum, A. C.: The hypertensive diabetic kidney as a model of the so-called collagen diseases. Canad. med. Ass. J. 88, 442—452 (1963).

Lutzner, M. A., J. H. Tierney, and and E. P. Benditt: Giant granules and widespread cytoplasmic inclusions in a genetic syndrome of Aleutian mink. Lab. Invest. 14, (12) 2063—2079 (1965).

OBEL, ANNA-LISA: Studies on a disease of mink with systemic proliferation of the plasma cells. Amer. J. vet. Res. 20, 384—393 (1959).

PADGETT, G. A., and E. O. DICKINSON: *In utero* death of feti in Aleutian disease. Nat. Fur News 37, 20—21 (1965).

PHILLIPS, L. L., and J. B. HENSON: Coagulation changes in Aleutian mink disease. Fed. Proc. 25, (2) Pt. 1, 620 (Abstract) (1966).

PORTER, D. D., and A. E. LARSEN: Statistical survey of Aleutian disease in ranch mink. Amer. J. vet. Res. 25, 1226—1229 (1964).

— F. J. DIXON, and A. E. LARSEN: Metabolism and function of gamma globulin in Aleutian disease of mink. J. exp. Med. 121, 889—900 (1965).

PROSE, P. H., L. LEE, and S. D. BALK: Electron microscopic study of the phagocytic fibrin-clearing mechanism. Amer. J. Path. 46, 3A — Scient. Proc. Amer. Assoc. Path. and Bact. (1965).

QUICK, A. J.: Hemorrhagic diseases. Philadelphia: Lea & Febiger, 1957.

QUIE, P. G., and J. G. HIRSCH: Antiserum to leucocyte lysosomes: its cytoxic, granulocytic and hemolytic activities. J. exp. Med. 120, 149—196 (1964).

RUBIN, H., L. FANSHIER, A. CORNELIUS, and W. F. HUGHES: Tolerance and immunity in chickens after congenital and contact infection with an avian leukosis virus. Virology 17, 143—156 (1962).

RUSSEL, J. D.: Research and control of Aleutian disease. Nat. Fur News 34, 8, 23, and 33 (1962).

SAISON, RUTH, L. KARSTAD, and T. J. PRIDHAM: Viral plasmacytosis (Aleutian disease) in mink. VI. The development of positive Coombs tests in experimental infections. Canad. J. comp. Med. 30, 151—156 (1966).

SIMON, G., and F. CHATELANAT: Fibrin and fibrinoid in the glomerulopathies. Comparative study in experimental and spontaneous pathology. Path. et Microbiol. (Basel) 26, (2), 191—205 (1963).

THOMPSON, G. R., and P. ALIFERIS: A clinical-pathological study of Aleutian mink disease; an experimental model for study of the connective-tissue diseases. Arthr. and Rheum. 7, 521—533 (1964).

THORMAR, H.: Neutralization of visna virus by antiserum from sheep. J. Immunol. 90, 185 (1963).

TRAUTWEIN, G.: Experimentelle Untersuchungen über die Aleutenkrankheit ("Aleutian disease") der Nerze. Arch. exp. Vet.-Med. 81, 287—395 (1964).

WEISSMANN, G.: Lysosomes (a review). New Engl. J. Med. 273, 1084—1090 and 1143—1149 (1965).

Acknowledgement. These studies were supported in part by a grant from the Medical Research Council of Canada.

Cell-Virus Interactions in Tissue Cultures Infected with Visna and Maedi Viruses

HALLDÓR THORMAR

Departamento de Virologia, Instituto Venezolano de Investigaciones Científicas
Apartado 1827, Caracas, Venezuela

With 6 Figures

Introduction

Visna and maedi are slowly progressing virus diseases of sheep affecting the central nervous system and the lungs, respectively. THORMAR and PÁLSSON (1966) recently reviewed the clinical and pathologic aspects of these two diseases.

In 1957 a virus was isolated in sheep choroid plexus tissue culture from a sheep brain showing lesions of visna (SIGURDSSON et al., 1960), and in 1958 a virus was isolated from the lungs of sheep affected with maedi in the same tissue culture system (SIGURDARDÓTTIR and THORMAR, 1964). Since then, these viruses have been isolated routinely from organs of sheep affected with visna and maedi. Tissue culture passages of the visna and maedi viruses consistently produce the respective disease in inoculated sheep. The viruses can be re-isolated from blood, cerebrospinal fluid, brain, lungs, and other organs of the animals during the preclinical as well as during the clinical phase of the diseases.

A comparison of visna and maedi viruses has shown that they are similar with respect to their physical, chemical, and biological characteristics (THORMAR, 1966a, 1966b). The viruses cross-react in neutralization tests, but antiserum against visna virus usually neutralize maedi virus to a lesser extent than the homologous virus strain (THORMAR and HELGADÓTTIR, 1965). All studies of visna and maedi viruses were conducted in monolayer cultures of choroid plexus cells of sheep. These cells are fibroblast-like and can be maintained through at least 20 serial passages.

Physical and Chemical Properties of the Viruses

Visna virus is medium sized. In osmium fixed preparations embedded in methacrylate the diameter of the virus particles varies between approximately 70 and 100 mµ, with an average of 85mµ. The particles are apparently spherical bodies surrounded by a thin membrane and containing a dense centrally located core, about 30 to 40 mµ in diameter. Similar particles were observed both in sections of infected cell cultures (THORMAR, 1961) and in sections of pellets sedimented by ultracentrifugation from tissue culture fluid with a titer of about 10^9 $TCID_{50}$ per ml (THORMAR and BIRCH-ANDERSEN, 1962 unpubl.).

In preparations stained with phosphotungstate the visna virus particles also vary considerably in size but generally appear larger than in methacrylate embedded preparations, being about 90 to 100 mµ in diameter. The particles are sur-

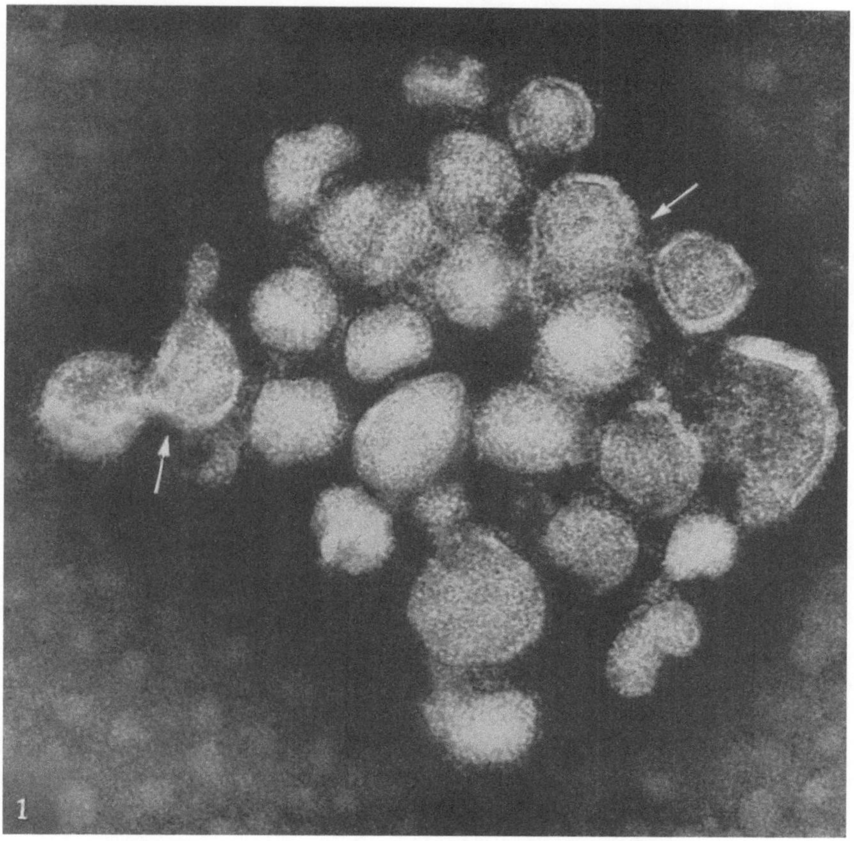

Fig. 1. A clump of visna virus particles. A concentric ring structure is indicated in the interior of some of the particles (arrows). Negative staining with potassium phosphotungstate, pH 7.0. Magnification: x 110,000. Reprinted from THORMAR and CRUICKSHANK. (Academic Press) Virology **25**, 145 (1965)

rounded by an envelope covered with projections measuring about 100 A in length and resembling the spikes which cover the envelope of influenza viruses (THORMAR and CRUICKSHANK, 1965). It has not yet been possible to detect with certainty the internal structure of the particles, but in a few instances a concentric ring arrangement was observed, suggesting a helical structure (Fig. 1).

Visna virus is rapidly inactivated at and below pH 4.2 and by heating at 56° C. It is sensitive to ether, chloroform, ethanol, phenol, metaperiodate, and trypsin. The virus is inactivated by ultraviolet light, but about 10 times more slowly than NDV, poliovirus and herpes virus (THORMAR, 1960, 1965 a).

The nucleic acid composition of the visna virion is as yet unknown. When tested with erythrocytes of a variety of species under various conditions, the virus did not hemagglutinate or cause hemadsorption (THORMAR, 1965a).

Maedi virus is in the size range of 60 to 90 mμ when measured in osmium fixed preparations embedded in methacrylate. Its size is probably not significantly different from that of visna virus. The structure of maedi virus in methacrylate embedded preparations as well as its sensitivity to chemical and physical agents is identical to that of visna virus, except that it is slightly more acid sensitive (THORMAR, 1965a).

Cell-Virus Interactions during a Growth Cycle at 37° C

Little is known about the earliest phase of interaction between visna virus and its host cell regarding virus attachment and penetration. There is, however, some indirect evidence that the virus adsorbs rapidly to the cell surface. Using a small inoculum, adsorption of virus appeared to be almost complete within 1 hour and was complete within 2 hours. An adsorption period as short as 1 minute was sufficient to cause infection of some of the cultures (THORMAR, 1963a).

When a small dose of virus was mixed with an excess of neutralizing antiserum and inoculated into tissue culture immediately without incubation, the cell layer became infected (THORMAR, 1963b). This is indirect evidence of rapid adsorption of visna virus and suggests that the rate of virus adsorption to the cell surface, is more rapid than the rate of neutralization of the virus by antibody.

After inoculation of cell monolayers with approximately 10 to 20 $TCID_{50}$ of visna virus per cell there is a latent period of about 20 hours before the first progeny virus appears. The events taking place during this rather long latent period are almost completely unknown. We know, however, that if 70 μM (20 μg per ml) of 5-bromodeoxyuridine (BUDR), an inhibitor of normal DNA synthesis, is added to the cell layers 1 to 2 hours after inoculation there is a complete inhibition of virus multiplication and cytopathic effect (THORMAR, 1965b). The effect of BUDR decreases rapidly with time; that added later than 2 hours after inoculation has a lessened effect, and that added later than 8 hours after inoculation has no effect (Fig. 2). Incubation of cell layers with BUDR for 20 hours prior to inoculation and during the 1 hour adsorption period had no demonstrable effect on the virus replication if the inhibitor was removed by washing at the end of this period. On the other hand, if the inhibitor was applied for a 6 hour period early in the latent phase and then removed by washing, there was a marked delay of virus formation. Since BUDR inhibits visna virus production in concentrations as low as those known to suppress normal DNA synthesis and the inhibition is partly overcome by addition of thymidine, the data seem to indicate that there is a period of DNA synthesis, which is necessary for the production of infective visna virus. This period of DNA synthesis is initiated in the cells 1 to 2 hours after infection and is largely completed in less than 8 hours or about 15 to 20 hours before the formation of virus.

Actinomycin D also interfered with the replication of visna virus. Cell monolayers were exposed to actinomycin D in a concentration of 0.25 μg per ml for periods of two and one-half hours at various times during the viral growth cycle. At the end of the two and one-half hour periods the inhibitor was removed from the culture medium by washing and the cell layers were incubated with fresh medium. All cultures were harvested 38 hours after inoculation and titrated. Actinomycin was found to inhibit virus formation when added during the latent period. If it was added during the growth phase, 20 to 30 hours after inoculation, it was found to stop further production of infective virus almost immediately. The effect of treatment with actinomycin seemed to be reversible, however, since virus multiplication was observed in the cultures if they were incubated for 2 to 3 days rather than for 38 hours before being harvested. Also, when actinomycin was added to the monolayers 18 to 20 hours before inoculation, it had no effect on the

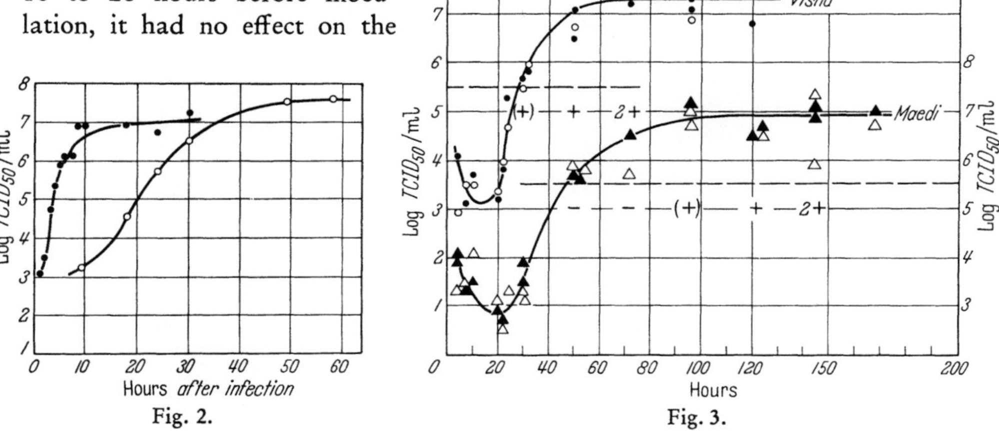

Fig. 2.   Fig. 3.

Fig. 2. Temporal relationship between inhibition by BUDR (●) and the growth cycle (○) of visna virus in monolayer cultures of sheep cells. BUDR was added to the cell cultures at various times after infection (abscissa) and the virus yield determined 58 hours after infection. Reprinted from THORMAR. (Academic Press) Virology 26, 36 (1965)

Fig. 3. Growth curves of visna and maedi viruses in monolayer cultures of sheep cells at 37° C. Free virus (●, ▲) and cell associated virus (○, △) is plotted against the time since inoculation. The horizontal broken lines indicate the approximate number of cells in the cultures. The degree of CPE is indicated by plus signs. Visna left and maedi right ordinate. Reprinted from THORMAR. Res. Vet. Sci. 6, 117 (1965)

yield of progeny virus measured 38 hours after inoculation. These experiments were interpreted to mean that visna virus reproduction depends on a DNA-directed RNA synthesis taking place shortly before the formation of the virus (THORMAR, 1965 b). The effect of BUDR and actinomycin D on the multiplication of visna virus seems to be similar to the effect of these inhibitors on the multiplication of Rous sarcoma virus as reported by TEMIN (1963, 1964) and by BADER (1964, 1965).

The growth phase of visna virus lasts about 15 to 20 hours (Fig. 3). Then virus production gradually levels off at about 100 TCID$_{50}$ per tissue culture cell. This figure represents the average minimum yield virus per host cell, since we do not know the actual number of infected cells in this system. Free virus in the fluid medium appears at about the same time as the cell associated virus (CAV), and during the growth phase the titer of free virus is equal or higher than that of CAV. The "release time" of visna virus was estimated by the method of Rubin and co-workers (1955) to be approximately 2 hours. Almost 99% of the CAV was neutralized by visna antiserum applied to the intact cell layer indicating that most of the virus was located at the cell membrane (Thormar, 1963a). It would appear,

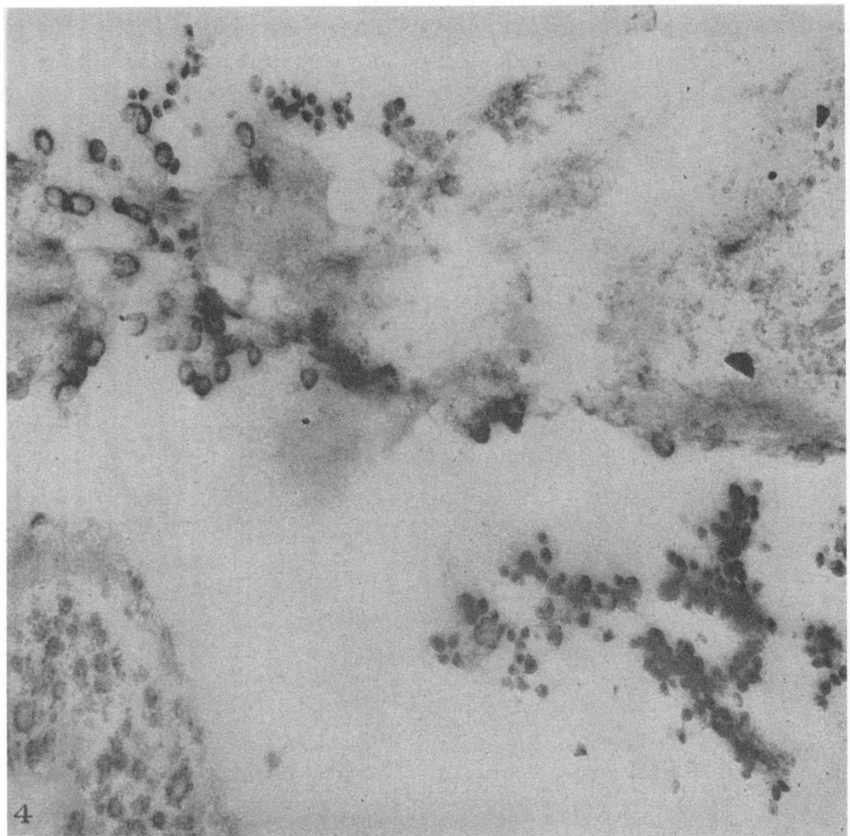

Fig. 4. A section of infected cells showing budding of the cell membrane, double-walled spherical bodies, and visna virus particles with a central core. OsO_4 fixation and lead hydroxide staining. Embedding in methacrylate. Magnification: ×18,000

therefore, that the infectious virus is formed at the time of its release from the cell. This is in accord with electron microscope studies of cell monolayers infected with visna virus which indicated that the virus particles were formed by budding of the external cell membrane and were released as double-walled spherical bodies (Figs. 4 and 5). After they separated from the cell, the double-walled bodies seemed to contract to form the typical visna virus particles which contain a central core bounded by an apparently single membrane. The double-walled bodies were always seen near cells showing budding of the cell membrane, and often they were mixed with the typical virus particles. Visna virus particles have not been observed intracellularly but were present in a large number outside the cells (THORMAR, 1961).

It is not known where in the host cells the various components of the visna virion are formed. Staining with acridine orange indicates that the structure of the nucleus is little affected by the infection, even in cells showing pronounced cytopathic effects (THORMAR, 1966c). The intensity of red fluorescence in the cytoplasm, on

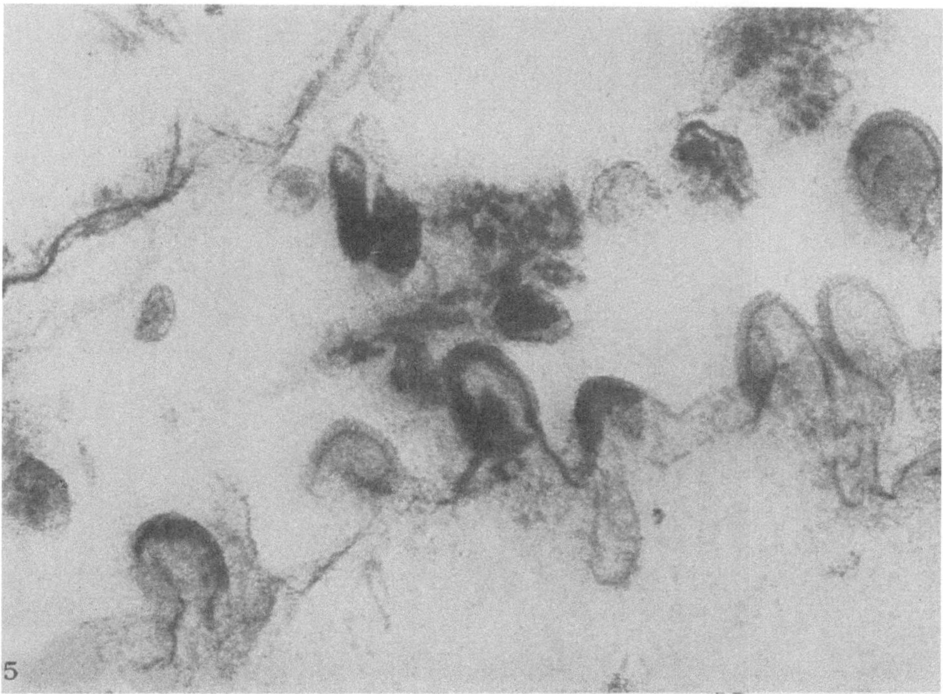

Fig. 5. A section of an infected cell showing budding of the cell membrane. Fixing, staining and embedding as in Fig. 4. Magnification: x 100,000

the other hand, is increased indicating an increased content of RNA. The stellate cells, characteristic for cell monolayers infected with visna virus, show bright red processes stretching out from the cytoplasm (Fig. 6). Increased green fluorescence, associated with an increased content of DNA, could not be detected either in the nucleus or in the cytoplasm. These observations indicate that RNA accumulates in the cytoplasm during the infection of the cells.

In cell cultures inoculated with a high dose of visna virus, i.e., about 10 to 20 $TCID_{50}$ per cell, the first CPE was visible about 25 to 30 hours after inoculation. Stellate cells with increased refractility were seen scattered near the margin of the cell layer. During the following 10 to 20 hours the CPE spread over the entire culture, converting most of the cells into large stellate forms. Shortly thereafter the cells rounded up and became separated from the glass. When cultures were fixed and stained, it was observed that the large stellate cells were multinucleated with 2 to at least 20 nuclei often arranged in a circle around the center of the giant cell (Siggurdsson et al., 1960). Increase in virus titer preceded the appearance of CPE and usually the titer reached its maximum before the degeneration of the cell layer began. It seemed likely, therefore, that infected cells released virus for a number of hours before they rounded up and degenerated.

Recently Harter and Choppin (1966, in press) demonstrated that large inocula of visna virus, i.e. greater than 20 $TCID_{50}$ per cell, caused an extensive syncytia formation in infected cell layers, appearing between 4 and 6 hours after inoculation. Virus multiplication was not necessary for this effect since it was also observed in cultures inoculated with virus which had been inactivated by ultraviolet light. The ability to cause cell fusion, therefore, seemed to be a property of the virus particle itself.

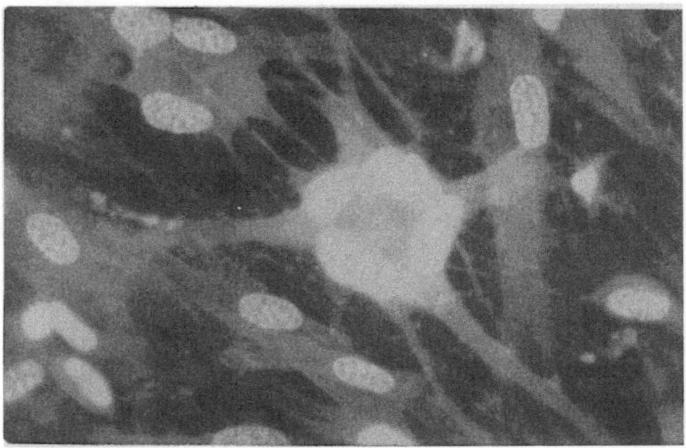

Fig. 6. Stellate cells from visna virus-infected monolayer stained with acridine orange

In cell layers inoculated with about 10 $TCID_{50}$ of maedi virus per cell, the first progeny virus appeared in about 30 hours (Fig. 3). The titer increased during the following 50 to 60 hours and levelled off about 4 days after inoculation at a value of about 50 $TCID_{50}$ of progeny virus per cell. At this time the first CPE was visible in the cell layer. Thus, the latent period was longer, the virus multiplication slower, and the CPE appeared much later than in cell cultures inoculated with the same amount of visna virus. The CPE of maedi virus was similar to that of visna virus, although there were not as many large stellate cells and more dense spindle-shaped cells with 2 or 3 nuclei and long cytoplasmic processes were noted. When large inocula are used, the CPE leads to complete destruction of the cell layer in 6 to 7 days.

Electron microscope studies showed that maedi virus was formed by budding at the external membrane of the host cells in the same manner as visna virus (Thormar, 1965a, 1966b).

Isolation and Growth in Tissue Cultures Containing Small Amounts of Virus

When small amounts of visna or maedi viruses were inoculated into monolayer cultures of choroid plexus cells, the appearance of CPE was delayed. The smallest detectable inoculum of visna virus produced CPE after about 12 to 14 days and the smallest inoculum of maedi virus after 16 to 20 days. Once a CPE appeared, however, complete disintegration of the cell layer developed within a few days.

In primary isolations of virus from sheep affected with visna or maedi the virus persisted in the cultures for months without ever completely destroying the cell layer. The technique used for virus isolation was to explant small pieces of tissue from an affected organ into a clot of chicken plasma in medium 199 with 20% sheep serum (SIGURDARDÓTTIR and THORMAR, 1964; SIGURDSSON et al., 1960). Outgrowths of cells from the explanted tissue were normally seen after 4 days, and during the following 3 to 5 days they formed a monolayer covering large areas of the glass surface. At this point the fluid medium was usually changed to medium 199 with 2% sheep serum. After a number of days, probably depending on the amount of virus present in the original explant, CPE appeared in the cell layer, and when the fluid was passed into fresh cell cultures it was found to contain small amounts of virus. The original cultures could be kept in the same roller tubes for as long as 4 to 5 months. During this time small amounts of virus were produced by the cell layer which showed a CPE with cell degeneration, but never disintegrated completely. If the concentration of normal sheep serum in the fluid medium was increased to 20%, an increased cell growth was observed and the partly destroyed cell layer was repaired and the CPE became less pronounced.

When the serum concentration was again reduced the CPE increased and the cell layer became discontinuous. Therefore, in these cultures a balance between cell growth and destruction of cells by the virus seemed to exist and this balance could be pushed in favor of cell growth, at least temporarily, by increasing the concentration of normal sheep serum. However, after a few passages in choroid plexus cultures the virus became adapted and caused complete cell degeneration within a limited time.

Discussion

Studies of the interactions between visna and maedi viruses and their host cells in tissue culture have not, so far, contributed greatly to our understanding of the extreme slowness of the infections caused by these viruses. Sheep become ill as late as 3 to 6 years after inoculation and apparently produce virus throughout all or most of the preclinical period as well as during the clinical phase of the disease (THORMAR and PÁLSSON, 1966). Probably many factors are involved, most of which have to be studied *in vivo*.

On the basis of the present data and data obtained by transmission experiments in sheep some factors may be suggested. Firstly, the visna and maedi virus infections in cell cultures can be considered as slow, even when large inocula of tissue culture adapted virus are used. When using very small inocula the time before the appearance of CPE is greatly prolonged and in explants from diseased organs the infection can be carried on in the same culture for months, since cell growth apparently can to some extent keep up with cell death. We do not know in which cells or tissues of the host animal the multiplication of visna and maedi viruses normally takes place, but since the primary histopathologic changes apparently are confined to the mesenchymal tissue of the central nervous system and the lungs, these tissues presumably are the site of infection and virus production. The histopathological changes consist mainly of proliferation of cells of the reticuloendothelial system, and an extensive infiltration, mostly of lymphocytes, plasma cells and microglia. This is seen particularly in visna without causing clinical illness. Therefore, visna and maedi infections seem to be caused by slowly growing viruses with a pronounced affinity for cell systems which can undergo considerable pathological change without the development of clinical signs. These factors together may account, at least partly, for the extremely long preclinical periods observed in visna and maedi.

The role of neutralizing antibody in visna and maedi infections is not yet understood. Circulating antibody does not prevent the spread of virus by the blood stream, probably because virus precursors are carried inside blood cells which protect them. The infected blood cells are able to release virus gradually, and since the rate of virus adsorption to the cell surface seems to be rapid compared with the rate of neutralization of virus by antibody, some of the released virus may be able to infect other cells.

Whether immunological reactions play a role in producing the histopathological lesions in visna and maedi is as yet completely unknown.

Summary

A review is given of studies of visna and maedi viruses in cell cultures, using strains of fibroblast-like cells from the choroid plexus of sheep brains.

Visna is a medium sized virus. It is spherical with a central core and bounded by a thin membrane. Staining with phosphotungstate has shown that the particles are surrounded by an envelope with projections similar to those of the influenza viruses. The virus is ether sensitive and is rapidly inactivated by heating to 56⁰ C. It does not hemagglutinate a variety of red cells tested under various conditions. Maedi virus is almost identical to visna virus in all properties studied.

After inoculation of about 10 to 20 $TCID_{50}$ of visna virus per cell into monolayer cell cultures there is a latent period of about 20 hours. If BUDR is added early in the latent period, it inhibits virus multiplication completely. If added 8 hours after inoculation it is almost without an effect on the later virus formation. Actinomycin D, on the other hand, is inhibitory to visna virus formation if added during the latent period or the growth phase, which lasts about 15 to 20 hours. During the growth phase the titer of free virus is equal to or greater than the titer of cell associated virus, and almost 99% of the cell associated virus can be neutralized by antiserum applied to the intact cell layer. Electron microscope studies have shown that the virus particles are formed by budding of the external cell membrane. Virus particles have not been observed inside the cells.

The growth cycle of maedi virus has been found to be slower than that of visna virus, the latent period being about 30 hours and the growth phase lasting for 2 to 3 days. When large inocula are used, a CPE of visna virus can be detected after 1 to 2 days and of maedi virus after about 4 days. When smaller inocula are used, the CPE appears after a longer time and the smallest detectable inoculum of tissue culture adapted virus causes CPE after 12 to 14 days (visna) or 16 to 20 days (maedi). In primary isolations of virus from sheep affected with visna or maedi, by explantation of tissue from affected organs into plasma clot, the virus can persist in the same culture for months without ever completely destroying the cell layer. The virus titer is low during all this period. After a few passages in a strain of choroid plexus cells the viruses become adjusted so that they cause a complete cell degeneration within a certain time. However, the visna and maedi virus infection in cell cultures can still be considered as slow, even when a large inoculum of tissue culture adapted virus is used.

References

BADER, J. P.: The role of deoxyribonucleic acid in the synthesis of Rous sarcoma virus. Virology **22**, 462—468 (1964).

— The requirement for DNA synthesis in the growth of Rous sarcoma and Rous-associated viruses. Virology **26**, 253—261 (1965).

HARTER, D. H., and P. W. CHOPPIN: Cell-fusing activity of a virus which causes a demyelinating disease. J. clin. Invest. (in press) (1966).

RUBIN, H., M. BALUDA, and J. E. HOTCHIN: The maturation of Western equine encephalomyelitis virus and its release from chick embryo cells in suspension. J. exp. Med. **101**, 205—212 (1955).

SIGURDARDÓTTIR, B., and H. THORMAR: Isolation of a viral agent from the lungs of sheep affected with maedi. J. infect. Dis. **114**, 55—60 (1964).

SIGURDSSON, B., H. THORMAR, and P. A. PÁLSSON: Cultivation of visna virus in tissue culture. Arch. ges Virusforsch. **10**, 368—381 (1960).

TEMIN, H. M.: The effects of actinomycin D on growth of Rous sarcoma virus in vitro. Virology **20**, 577—582 (1963).

— The participation of DNA in Rous sarcoma virus production. Virology **23**, 486—494 (1964).

THORMAR, H.: Stability of visna virus in infectious tissue culture fluid. Arch. ges. Virusforsch. **10**, 501—509 (1960).

— An electron microscope study of tissue cultures infected with visna virus. Virology **14**, 463—475 (1961).

— The growth cycle of visna virus in monolayer cultures of sheep cells. Virology **19**, 273—278 (1963 a).

— Neutralization of visna virus by antisera from sheep. J. Immunol. **90**, 185—192 (1963 b).

— A comparison of visna and maedi viruses. I. Physical, chemical and biological properties. Res. Vet. Sci. **6**, 117—129 (1965 a).

— Effect of 5-bromodeoxyuridine and actinomycin D on the growth of visna virus in cell cultures. Virology **26**, 36—43 (1965 b).

— Physical, chemical and biological properties of visna virus and its relationship to other animal viruses. In: Slow, latent and temperate virus infections, p. 335—340. Nat. Inst. Neurol. Dis. Blind. Monograph No. 2. U. S. Public Health Service (1966 a).

— A study of maedi virus. In: Proceedings of the International Conference on Lung Tumours in Animals, Perugia, p. 393—402 (1965, 1966 b).

— Observations on visna virus-infected cell cultures stained with acridine orange. Acta path. microbiol. scand. **68**, 54—58 (1966 c).

—, and A. BIRCH-ANDERSEN: Unpublished work.

Thormar, H., and J. G. Cruickshank: The structure of visna virus studied by the negative staining technique. Virology 25, 145—148 (1965).
—, and H. Helgadóttir: A comparison of visna and maedi viruses. II. Serological relationship. Res. Vet. Sci. 6, 456—465 (1965).
—, and P. A. Pálsson: Visna and maedi — two slow infections of sheep and their etiological agents. In: Perspectives in virology, vol. 5, Academic Press, 1966.

Immune and Autoimmune Reactions in the Pathogenesis of Slow Virus Disease*

John Hotchin

Division of Laboratories and Research,
New York State Department of Health,
and
Institute of Preventive Medicine, Albany Medical College
Albany, New York

With 7 Figures

The slow virus diseases are a fascinating example of an immunological enigma which may be at the center of the mechanism of slow virus disease pathogenesis. Studies on lymphocytic choriomeningitis (LCM) virus infection in mice showed that animals which had been inoculated at birth could suffer from a long continued infection with high titers of virus (Hotchin 1961, 1962). This "persistent tolerant infection" (PTI) (Hotchin and Weigand, 1961) was found to lead, after approximately 10 months, to a debilitating fatal disease (Hotchin, 1962; Hotchin and Collins, 1964). A brief look at this situation with LCM will introduce the main subject of my discussion.

Fig. 1 shows early results (Hotchin and Weigand, 1961) obtained by inoculation shortly after birth of LCM virus into mice of different ages. Intracerebral inoculation at any time between 4 and 7 days caused 100 per cent mortality. As the day of inoculation was moved closer to the time of birth, mortality dropped until at approximately 6 hours after birth it was below 20 per cent. For some unexplained reason inoculation earlier than 6 hours caused a higher rate of mortality. The curve relating mortality to age at inoculation has the same general shape as those curves relating the degree of effectiveness of induction of acquired immunological tolerance following inoculation of tissue cells. Presumably the mechanisms are similar if not the same. If one observes those inoculated mice which survive for long periods of time after such neonatal infection, one finds that regardless of the time of inoculation, there is continuing high level virus infection with high titers in the blood for many months after inoculation. Table 1 shows a few representative titers taken 195 days after intracerebral inoculation within a few days of birth

* This investigation was supported (in part) by research grant AI-03846 from the National Institutes of Health, United States Public Health Service.

(HOTCHIN, 1962). It seems that in persistent tolerant infection with LCM virus, we have a unique situation in which a virus infection is continuously active at a high level during the life span of the affected animal, a crucially important factor in slow virus disease which is worth comparing with standard virological latency.

The main factors in establishing latent and persistent tolerant infections with virus are compared in Table 2. The most important one in establishing the PTI state is the level of virus titer in the affected animal; in "ordinary" latency this is low or minimal, and it may be difficult to find evidence of active virus at all, whereas in the PTI state the titer is high and comparable to titers found at the peak of acute virus disease. Concomitantly there exists an inverse situation regarding antiviral antibody, since in the PTI state no neutralizing antibody is ordinarily detectable whereas definite antibody is found in latency as, for example, with herpes simplex virus (SCOTT and TOKUMARU, 1965). The nature of the virus also differs in that it may be masked by antibody in laten-

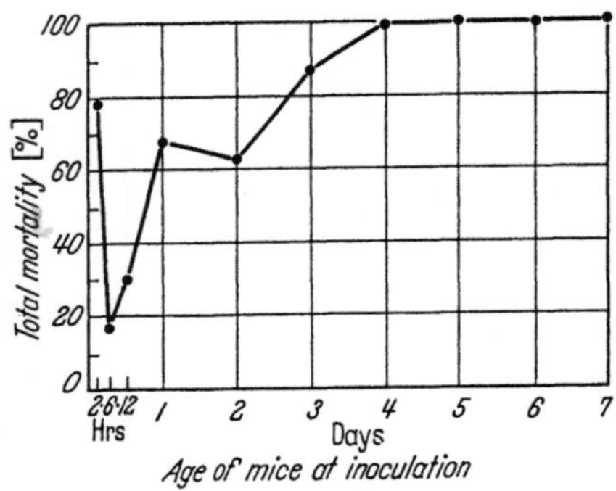

Fig. 1. The relationship between mortality and age at inoculation of infant mice with LCM virus

cy, whereas in PTI animals at least a high proportion of the virus is in the free or unmasked state. Nonspecific agents (SCOTT and TOKUMARU, 1965) and immuno-suppressive drugs (GOTTMANN and BEATTY, 1962) can activate latent virus infections such as herpes, cytomegalovirus and varicella to a higher level of virus titer and activity while they have no effect on the PTI state (HOTCHIN, 1962; HOTCHIN and CINITS, 1958), which therefore takes on the attributes of a special condition, differing in important respects from latency.

Mice which have been made PTI with certain strains of LCM virus exhibit a slow virus disease after an incubation period of approximately 10 months (HOTCHIN, 1962; HOTCHIN and COLLINS,

Table 1. *Pooled blood titers of PTI mice 195 days after inoculation*

Age when inoculated with virus	LD$_{50}$/ml blood
2 hours	$10^{4.7}$
12 hours	$10^{4.6}$
4 days	$10^{4.2}$
6 days	$10^{4.2}$

1964). Fig. 2 depicts a mortality curve due to late onset disease (LD) in female mice. Four groups of animals are shown, consisting of the experimental group (PTI) which received neonatal IC inoculation with LCM virus, and three control groups which received normal mouse liver, no inoculation, or LCM virus inoculation given subcutaneously at 1 month of age. After approximately 10 months the mortality of the PTI group rose sharply, reaching approximately 90 per cent by 20 months after inoculation, whereas all control groups were very much below this. The reason for the temporary upsurge of mortality in the normal mouse liver-inoculated group is at present unknown. The same results were obtained with male mice, although the picture was less clear because these animals tend to have a higher background mortality due to fighting. LCM virus thus offers an example of a slow virus disease which results only if the agent is introduced neonatally with consequent production of immunological tolerance.

Table 2. *Comparison of latent and persistent tolerant infections*

Factor	Latency	PTI
Virus titer	Low	High
Antibody	Present	Absent
Virus	Masked	Unmasked (free)
X-ray, UVL, etc.	Activate	—
Immunosuppressive drugs	Activate	—

Other known or candidate slow virus diseases may be compared as to possible methods of pathogenesis. Table 3 lists some slow virus diseases of animals, including those capable of causing disease after inoculation of adult animals and those requiring neonatal or congenital infection. The host species is shown and also the main site or "target organ" of pathology. Scrapie is listed under both

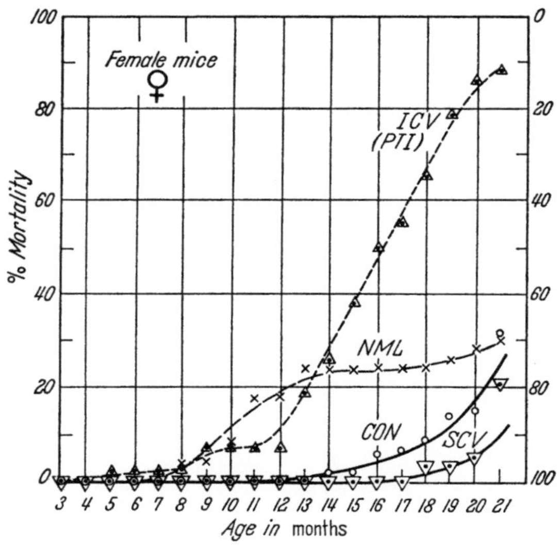

Fig. 2. The relationship between cumulative mortality and time, in four groups of female mice. ICV = mice received LCM mouse liver IC at one day of age. NML = mice received normal mouse liver IC at one day of age. CON = mice received no inoculation. SCV = mice received LCM virus (same dose as ICV) at one month of age, by the SC route

categories since this infection can apparently be congenital or acquired later in life. Lactic dehydrogenase-elevating or serum enzyme-elevating virus so far is known to affect only the enzyme levels of the blood and does not produce any other disease or pathology (NOTKINS et al., 1963); however, observation of affected mice may yet reveal a slow virus disease, although at present this agent could be considered to cause essentially an incubation period without a subsequent

Table 3. *Slow virus diseases of animals*

Disease agent	Animals	Target organ
Adult :		
Scrapie } Rida }	Sheep	Cerebellum
Plasmacytosis (Aleutian disease)	Mink	Connective tissue
African swine fever	Swine	Lungs
Encephalopathy of mink	Mink	Cerebellum
Visna (Maedi)	Sheep	CNS
Infectious adenomatosis	Sheep	Lungs
Trifur equorum (equine infectious anemia)	Horses	Blood cells
Congenital :		
Scrapie	Sheep	Cerebellum
LDH	Mice	Blood enzymes
SMCA	Mice	?CNS
LCM	Mice	Kidney (multiple)

disease. Suckling mouse cataract agent not only induces cataracts after neonatal inoculation but also causes minor neurological changes in the mice.

Comparable conditions of man, some of which are included on a tentative basis, are listed in Table 4. Serum hepatitis is included here as possible example of persistent tolerant infection. Persisting congenital infection with this virus in

Table 4. *Slow virus disease of man (tentative)*

Disease agent	Target organ
Adult :	
Serum hepatitis	Liver
Kuru	Cerebellum
?Multiple sclerosis	CNS
?Amyotrophic lateral sclerosis	CNS
Aleutian mink disease	Connective tissue
Equine infectious anemia	Blood cells
?Iceland disease	CNS
?Motor neuron disease of New Guinea	CNS
Congenital :	
Serum hepatitis	Liver? multiple

man would be an excellent human parallel to the LCM-PTI mouse model. It has been proposed as a candidate for inclusion as a persistent tolerant infection several times (Hotchin, 1962; Hotchin and Collins, 1964; Hotchin, 1958). Recently Burnet has speculated that it can induce chronic hepatitis after several years, and also that it may be the cause of kuru in New Guinea (Mathews, 1965). However, it seems likely that the kuru agent isolated by GAJDUSEK, GIBBS and ALPERS (1966) is a separate entity and not the virus of serum hepatitis. Russian workers claim to have isolates for both multiple sclerosis and amyotrophic lateral sclerosis (ZILBER et al., 1963). Human cases of both Aleutian mink disease (CHAPMAN and JIMMEZ, 1963) and equine infectious anemia have been recorded (PETERS, 1954). Iceland disease, although of dubious status as a slow virus agent, does cause long-continued after-effects for as many as 6 years (SIGURDSSON and GUDMIENDSSON, 1956) involving tenderness, pain and nervousness, all symptoms which might be considered psychological if this agent had not caused outbreaks on epidemic scale. GAJDUSEK (1963) has described a motor-neuron disease in natives of New Guinea which has similarities to kuru and, like it, may prove to be a slow virus disease. Rubella virus

Table 5. *Relation between age and positive virus isolation in infants cultured serially for rubella virus*

Age in months	Ratio of positive infants to total cultured	Percentage positive
0–1	13/17	77
2–3	6/11	55
4–5	3/11	25
>6	0/9	0

almost qualifies as causing a persistent tolerant infection of man, but the duration of this is only a few months after birth, presumably constituting only a half-stage toward the PTI state. Table 5 shows some information on the persistence of rubella virus (LINDQUIST et al., 1965) which is somewhat reminiscent of the LCM situation in mice. The virus can persist in human infants for approximately 6 months after birth before the immune system of the affected child is able finally to eliminate it.

Since the persistence of active virus replication appears so crucial in slow virus disease, a survey of the more obvious examples for their properties may be relevant to this concept. Table 6 lists the available data from current literature. Many of the agents listed persist for long periods involving months or years. This is true for scrapie (HADLOW, 1961; EKLUND et al., 1963; J. GIBBS, personal communication), encephalopathy of mink (HARTSOUGH and BURGER, 1965; BURGER and HARTSOUGH, 1965)which may well prove to be the same agent as scrapie, and rida (ZLOTNIK and KATIYAR, 1961), which is regarded as scrapie occurring in Iceland; also it is true for suckling mouse cataract agent (CLARK, 1964), the lactic dehydrogenase virus (RILEY, 1963; BAILEY et al., 1963; RILEY et al., 1965), and African swine fever (DEBOER, 1966). The latter virus (DEBOER, 1966) causes a persistent tolerant infection in pigs which can apparently (DEBOER, personal communication) cause a fatal slow virus disease of the lung. This virus disease appears to provide an almost exact duplication of the LCM-PTI-LD situation in mice. According to ZILBER et al. (1963), ALS falls in the same category of slow virus disease; and visna has been shown by the work of SIGURDSSON et al. (1957); SIGURDSSON and PÁLSSON (1958); THORMAR and GUDNADÓTTIR (in press) to persist for years, as does the kuru agent

(GAJDUSEK et al., 1966). Equine infectious anemia virus persists for a long time (FRIEDMAN, 1964), as does serum hepatitis virus in man (HAVENS and PAUL, 1965). Information concerning antibody production is somewhat scattered but, when available, is strongly in favor of these agents, which are for some reason poor inducers of neutralizing antibody. To date there is no evidence that antibody to scrapie can be made (J. GIBBS, personal communication), either in the affected animal or in alternative hosts; and in the case of visna the Icelandic workers have shown (THORMAR, 1966) that sometimes several years elapse before antibody finally appears.

Table 6. *A comparison of immunological properties of slow viruses*

Virus	Long incubation period (Months or years)	Poor, very late or absent antibody	Persistent virus in organs
Scrapie (Rida) (11, 6, 22)	+	+	+
Aleutian mink disease (12, 34, 15)	+	+	+
Encephalopathy of mink (13, 2)	+	+	+
SMCA (4)	+ ?		+
LDH (27, 1, 28)	+ ?	+	+
African swine fever (5)	+	+	+
Visna (Maedi) (32, 33, 35)	+	+	+
Kuru (9)	+		+
Equine infectious anemia (7)	+	+	+
Serum hepatitis (14)	+	+	+

From these observations the following tentative conclusions have been reached concerning the general properties of slow viruses: (1) They actively multiply to high titers in the host for long periods of time without apparent disease. (2) These viruses are not recognized as "foreign" by the host, perhaps because they possess antigenic constitutions relatively similar to that of the host or perhaps because they produce a direct effect upon the host immune tissue. (3) An immune reaction to such tolerated agents either is very late or does not occur at all. (4) The final disease produced may be an autoimmune response caused by termination of the tolerance, although the final disease may be agradual process of "erosion" of the affected cells by the virus.

From these ideas a working concept for a practical approach to the further study of slow virus pathogenesis is as follows: Because the host finds great difficulty in recognizing these viruses as foreign, the PTI state is a fundamental prerequisite for slow virus disease. The long continued PTI state allows a time-dependent event to occur during the ensuing long "incubation period". Thus the slow virus diseases are slow, not necessarily because of intrinsic slowless of the viral agent in replication or spread as has been clearly shown, e.g. for LCM (HOTCHIN, 1962) and scrapie (EKLUND et al., 1963), but because of some special interaction between the virus and the host. This "time bomb" effect is presumably mediated either by a virus tissue reaction in the infected cells or possibly via an immunological factor such as the gradual appearance and selection of a mutant clone.

At the present time the pathogenesis of the slow virus diseases may be considered from two major points of view. The first is the antigen-antibody problem, centering around the question of the mechanism of tolerance induction and lack

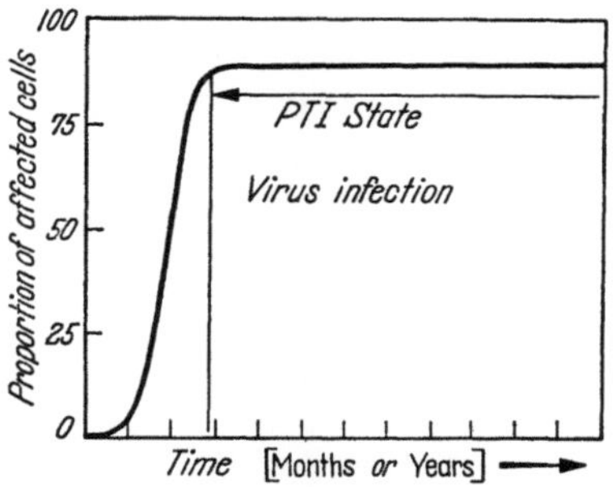

Fig. 3. The relationship between the proportion of virus infected susceptible cells and time in a hypothetical model slow virus system

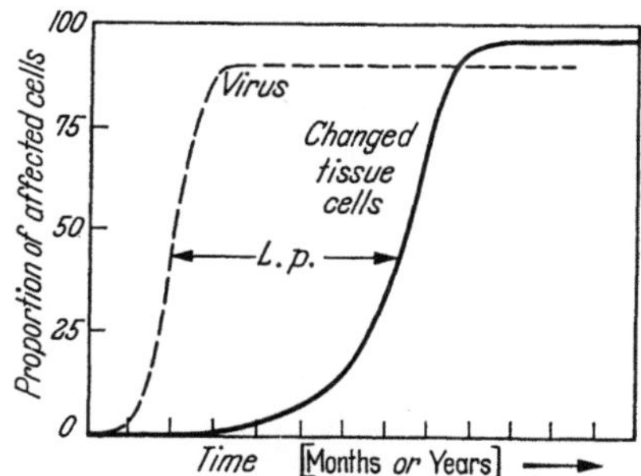

Fig. 4. The relationship between the proportion of changed tissue cells and time, in a hypothetical model slow virus system

of neutralizing antibody response, and the second concerns the problem of the very gradual or late tissue damaging effect. From these viewpoints consideration of an imaginary model slow virus disease from a theoretical point of view is in order. Fig. 3 shows a curve relating the proportion of infected cells to the passage of time after inoculation of the host by the slow virus. The ordinate represents the

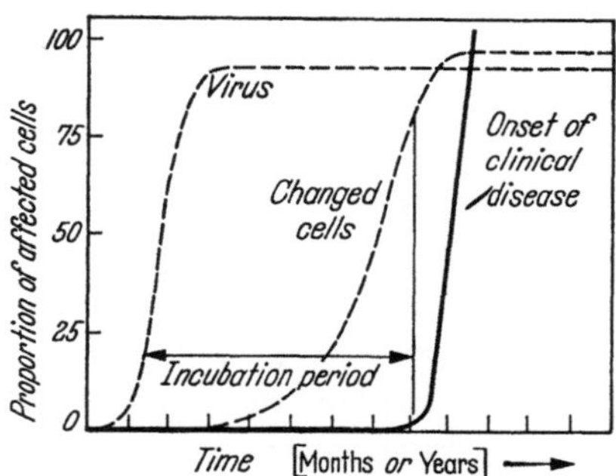

Fig. 5. The relationship between the onset of clinical disease and time in a hypothetical model slow virus system

porportion of cells which are important in the disease, i.e., the "target organ". Examples of this occur in the cerebellar cells in scrapie or kuru. Mere infection of the cells presumably does not of itself cause any damage or sign of disease. After this period the situation remains constant during the persisting tolerant infection until the expiration of a latent period shown as l. p. on Fig. 4. In this diagram the previous curve is shown as a dotted line; the solid line now represents the increase in the proportion of changed or damaged tissue cells, as a result of the virus activity. The damage is a final consequence either of virus growth in the cells themselves or a consequence of an immunological attack on the virus infected tissue. In Fig. 5

these data are again portrayed in the dotted form; in addition the solid line now represents the development of clinical signs of disease with respect to time, based on the assumption that these will become manifest only after a certain critical proportion of functionally essential cells has been seriously damaged. In this example, such a level is taken as 75 per cent; a perpendicular dropped from this point on the changed cell curve would intersect the abscissa at the time of onset of clinical disease, as shown in Fig. 5. Under these conditions the time interval between this perpendicular and the first curve (Fig. 3) is equal to the incubation period of the disease. The rate of development of full-blown clinical disease under these conditions may be expected to be very rapid, since the changed cell curve will

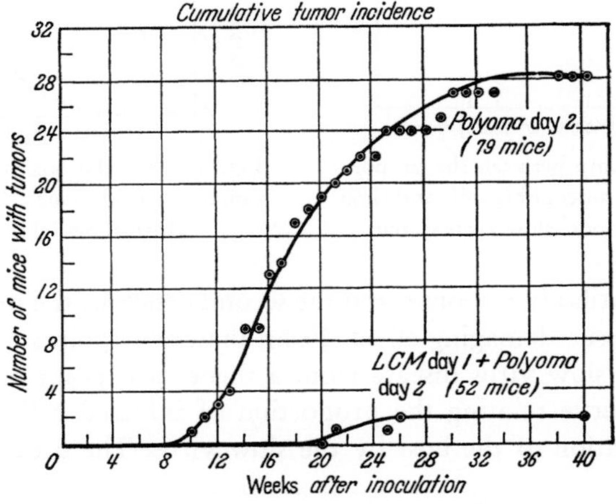

Fig. 6. The relationship between polyoma virus induced tumor production and time in groups of mice inoculated one or two days after birth

pass from 75 to 100 per cent in a relatively short time and the functional impairment of the target organ is likely to have had a fatal result before all cells are decayed.

This hypothesis of the pathogenesis of slow virus disease is a fairly simple and obvious one but it does not explain the long latent period, the exact cause of which may remain elusive for a correspondingly long time. However, the tumor viruses, which should technically be included in the slow virus group, suggest a possible mechanism for "time bomb" or latent period effect. The time interval between inoculation and clinical disease with these agents is a close parallel to that for the slow viruses. The main difference between the two groups is that the tumor viruses cause a transformation which produces an obvious local result, i. e., a tumor. If the other slow viruses also produce non-tumorous transformations at about the same rate, these may well be responsible for the cellular damage caused either by functional impairment or via a new cellular surface antigen. The latter would then presumably evoke an immune response resulting in autoimmune cellular destruction. The rate of transformation of cells by a tumor virus might correspond to the rate of slow virus transformation. Such data are available in terms of the rate of development of tumors in a population of polyoma virus inoculated mice. This result was obtained in the course of some earlier experiments (HOTCHIN, 1962) on the effects of persistent tolerant infection with LCM virus upon tumor induction by polyoma virus; during this work a remarkable suppressive effect of LCM virus was observed which is shown in Fig. 6. In this figure the suppressive effect shown by the LCM virus is of lesser interest than the shape of the curve relating tumor incidence to time. This curve can be regarded as an

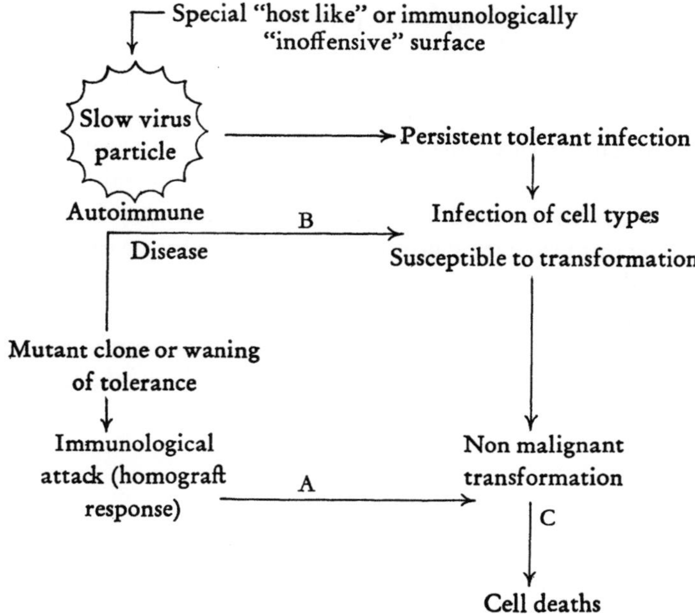

A, B, and C are alternative mechanisms which result in destruction of specific target tissues.

Fig. 7. In this diagram the slow virus is seen as having special surface properties whereby it is either host-like in its antigenic structure or somehow inoffensive in an immunological sense and thereby able to induce persistent tolerant infection. Subsequently the long continued PTI state allows infection of special cell types which are subjected to cell death either as a direct result of the virus induced transformation or change, or possibly mediated by an immune response directed against new cellular antigens

indication of the rate of appearance of cellular manifestations of the long term effects of a slow virus. It was clear from the clinical observation of the rate of increase in size of the tumors that this was a very rapid affair and was short (about 3 weeks) relative to the period during which tumors appeared (26 weeks); this interval could not significantly affect the shape of the curve of which the main determinant was the latent period involved in the transformation process and the initiation of tumor growth. Therefore a close similarity exists between the shape of this curve which was found by direct observation of an *in vivo* situation and the curve (Fig. 4) representing changed cells in the hypothetical model of slow virus pathogenesis. At the present time, tumor transformation is the only virus induced cell transformation with a visible marker—the tumor; therefore it is at present not possible to tell whether the other slow viruses also induce transformations which though non-malignant nevertheless derange the cell sufficiently to cause loss of function; perhaps the mere accumulation of viral material, as suggested by Johnson (in press), is enough for this. This hypothesis of slow virus pathogenesis can be summarized as follows (Fig. 7): Slow viruses multiply for a long period of time in the host with access to virtually all types of cell. Infection of certain cell types is followed after a long latent period by non-malignant transformation (or other change) of these cells which, possibly aided by immune attack, results in loss of function; when the functional reserves of the tissue are exhausted, clinical disease ensues.

The above concept of slow virus disease is necessarily a tentative one, but it may be hoped that it has the merit of being open to several experimental approaches, particularly in the field of immunology, which may lead to new information concerning this fascinating group of viruses. Twelve years ago, Sigurdsson (1954) who coined the term "slow infection", summed up the situation when he said: "If there is a group of slow virus infections with a number of fundamental characteristics in common, as I have suggested, it might be helpful for us to realize this. If there is a 'basic theme' running through these slow infections, we should try to discover it."

References

Bailey, J. M., M. Stearman and J. Clough: LDH levels in blood and tissues of mice infected with an LDH agent. Proc. Soc. exp. Biol. (N. Y.) 114, 148 (1963).

Burger, D., and G. R. Hartsough: Encephalopathy of mink. II. Experimental and natural transmission. J. infect. Dis. 115, 393 (1965).

Chapman, I., and F. A. Jimmez: Aleutian-mink disease in man. New Engl. J. Med. 269, 1171 (1963).

Clark, H. F.: Suckling mouse cataract agent. J. infect. Dis. 114, 476 (1964).

DeBoer, C. J.: Studies to determine neutralizing antibody in sera from animals recovered from African swine fever and laboratory animals inoculated with African swine fever virus with adjuvants. Fed. Proc. 25, (2) part 1, 615 (1966).

Eklund, C. M., W. J. Hadlow, and R. C. Kennedy: Some properties of the scrapie agent and its behavior in mice. Proc. Soc. exp. Biol. (N. Y.) 112, 974 (1963).

Friedman, J. C. L'anémie infectieuse des équidés. Nouv. Rev. franç. Hémat. 4, 421 (1964).

Gajdusek, D. C.: Motor-neuron disease in natives of New Guinea. New Engl. J. Med. 268, 474 (1963).

— C. J. Gibbs, Jr., and M. Alpers: Experimental transmission of a kurulike syndrome to chimpanzees. Nature (Lond.) 209, 794 (1966).

Gottman, A. W., and E. C. Beatty Jr.: Cytomegalic inclusion disease in children with leukemia or lymphosarcoma. Amer. J. Dis. Child. 104, 180 (1962).

Hadlow, W. J.: The pathology of experimental scrapie in the dairy goat. Res. Vet. Sci. 2, 289 (1961).

Hartsough, G. R., and J. R. Gorham: Aleutian disease in mink. Nat. Fur News 28, 10 (1956).

—, and D. Burger: Encephalopathy of mink. 1. Epizootiologic and clinical observations. J. infect. Dis. 115, 387 (1965).

HAVENS, W. P., and J. R. PAUL: Infectious hepatitis and serum hepatitis. In: Viral and rickettsial infections of man (HORSFALL and TAMM, ed.). Philadelphia: J. B. LIPPINCOTT Co. 1965.

HENSON, J. B., R. W. LEADER, and J. R. GORHAM: Hypergamma globulinemia in mink. Proc. Soc. exp. Biol. (N. Y.) **107**, 919 (1961).

HOTCHIN, J. E.: Some aspects of induced latent infection of mice with the virus of lymphocytic choriomeningitis. In: Symposium on Latency and Masking in Viral and Rickettsial Infections. Wisconsin Medical School, Madison, Sept. 4, 5, and 6, 1957. Minneapolis: Burgess Publ. Co. 1958.

— The role of immunological tolerance in neonatal infection of mice with lymphocytic choriomeningitis virus. Quart. Rev. Pediat. **16**, 97 (1961).

— The biology of lymphocytic choriomeningitis infection: Virus-induced immune disease. Cold Spr. Harb. Symp quant Biol. **27**, 479 (1962).

—, and M. CINITS: Lymphocytic choriomeningitis infection of mice as a model for the study of latent virus infection. Canad. J. Microbiol. **4**, 149 (1958).

—, and D. N. COLLINS: Glomerulonephritis and late onset disease of mice following neonatal virus infection. Nature (Lond.) **203**, 1357 (1964).

—, and H. WEIGAND: Studies of lymphocytic choriomeningitis in mice. J. Immunol. **86**, 392 (1961).

JOHNSON, R. T.: Pathways of invasion and spread. Symposium on Chronic Infectious Neuropathic Agent (CHINA) ("Slow" virus infections). In press.

LINDQUIST, J. M., S. A. PLOTKIN, L. SHAW, R. V. GUDEN, and M. L. WILLIAMS: Congenital rubella syndrome as a systemic infection. Studies of Affected Infants Born in Philadelphia, U. S. A. Brit. Med. J. **1965** II, 1401.

MATHEWS, J. D.: The changing face of kuru. Lancet **1965** I, 1138.

NOTKINS, A. L., R. E. GREENFIELD, D. MARSHALL, and L. BANE: Multiple enzyme changes in the plasma of normal and tumor-bearing mice following infection with the lactic dehydrogenase agent. J. exp. Med. **117**, 185 (1963).

PETERS, J. T.: Trifur equorum infection in man. New Engl. J. Med. **251**, 1022 (1954).

RILEY, V.: Enzymatic determination of transmissible replicating factors associated with mouse tumors. Ann. N. Y. Acad. Sci. **100**, 762 (1963).

— J. D. LOVELESS, M. A. FITZMAURICE, and W. M. SILVER: Mechanism of lactate dehydrogenase (LDH) elevation in virus-infected hosts. Life Sci. **4**, 487 (1965).

SCOTT, T. F M., and T. TOKUMARU: The herpes virus group. In: Viral and rickettsial infections of man (HORSFALL and TAMM, ed.), Philadelphia: J. B. Lippincott Co. 1965.

SIGURDSSON, B.: Rida: A chronic encephalitis of sheep with general remarks on infections which develop slowly and some of their special characteristics. Brit. vet. J. **110**, 341 (1954).

—, and K. GUDMIENDSSON: Clinical findings six years after outbreak of akureyri disease. Lancet **1956** I, 766.

— P. A. PÁLSSON, and H. GRÍMSON: Visna, a demyelinating transmissible disease of sheep. J. Neuropath. exp. Neurol. **16**, 389 (1957).

— — Visna of sheep. A slow, demyelinating infection. Brit. J. exp. Path. **39**, 519 (1958).

THOMPSON, G. R., and P. ALIFERIS: A clinical-pathological study of Aleutian mink disease, an experimental model for study of the connective-tissue diseases. Arthr. and Rheum. **7**, 521 (1964).

THORMAR, H.: Visna and Maedi — two slow infections of sheep and their etiological agents. In press (1966).

ZIL'BER, L. A., Z. L. BAJDAKOVA, A. N. GARDAS'JAN, N. V. KONOVALOV, T. L. BUNINA, and E. M. BARABADZE: Study of the etiology of amyotrophic lateral sclerosis. Bull. Wld Hlth Org. **29**, 449 (1963).

ZLOTNIK, I., and R. D. KATIYAR: The occurrence of scrapie disease in sheep of the remote Himalayan foothills. Vet. Rec. **73**, 543 (1961).

Search for Infectious Etiology in Chronic and Subacute Degenerative Diseases of the Central Nervous System

Clarence J. Gibbs, Jr.

Laboratory of Slow, Latent, and Temperate Virus Infections,
National Institute of Neurological Diseases and Blindness,
National Institutes of Health, Bethesda, Md.

Our interest in slow infections stems from the early work of Gajdusek and Zigas (1957) which provided the first description of a strange new subacute, familial, degenerative disease of the central nervous system, characterized by cerebellar ataxia and trembling, called "Kuru" by the New Guineans who suffer from it. This disease, restricted to some 12,000 natives of the Fore linguistic group indigenous to the Eastern Highlands of New Guinea and to their immediate neighbors with whom they intermarry, accounted for over half of the total deaths that have occurred in their population (Gajdusek and Zigas, 1957; Gajdusek, 1963). The disease was first suspected to be a meningoencephalitis. However, the lack of detectable febrile response, absence of cerebrospinal fluid pleocytosis, the general lack of an elevated protein content and the absence of extensive perivascular cuffing or other neuropathological reactions typical of infectious processes did not support the possibility of an acute infectious etiology. Further, the epidemiological pattern of Kuru, restricting its spread in peripheral areas to individuals who are genetically related to the population in the center of the endemic region, suggested some genetic determinent of disease expression. The early hypothesis that the disease might be due to an auto-sensitization reaction was not borne out by neuropathology or by the search for autoimmune antibodies to brain antigen in serum specimens.

In 1959 Hadlow reported close similarities between the neuropathology, clinical symptoms, and epidemiology of Kuru in man and of scrapie in sheep. Scrapie is a slowly progressive degenerative disease of the central nervous system, with an infectious etiology, to which susceptibility was shown to be genetically determined (Gordon, 1946; Stamp, 1958). The disease in sheep tends to run an afebrile course with a long incubation period of from 2 to 5 years. There is no cerebrospinal fluid pleocytosis or increase in protein content, and the neuropathological changes usually attendant in viral infections of the nervous system are not evident. Thus, the entire problem of an infectious etiology for Kuru had to be reconsidered in the light of slow infections. This same approach would certainly be effective in work on other subacute and chronic nervous system degenerations such as multiple sclerosis, subacute inclusion body encephalitis, Parkinson's disease, amyotrophic lateral sclerosis and the related amyotrophic lateral sclerosis-Parkinsonism dementia syndrome seen in the Chamorro people in the Mariana Islands, and the Werdnig-Hoffman disease, to illustrate a few representative diseases. All previous attempts to isolate transmissible agents from these human diseases would certainly have been unsuccessful using techniques applied to acute self-limited viral infections. Rarely did investigators maintain inoculated experimental animals under observation for periods of from three to five years as may at times be necessary for clinical manifestation of scrapie in naturally infected sheep, of visna and maedi infections in sheep, of scrapie-like disease reported as occurring only in Icelandic sheep inoculated with human brain from an unusual type of multiple sclerosis (PÁLSSON et al., 1965), and of an experimentally induced amyotrophic lateral sclerosis-like syndrome observed in monkeys and reported by ZILBER in the U.S.S.R.

Thus, in 1962 we reinitiated attempts to transmit to animals Kuru and a number of other degenerative diseases of the central nervous system. We employed scrapie as a model, keeping in mind SIGURDSSON's criteria for slow infections: (a) a long initial period of latency lasting from several months to several years; (b) a regular protracted course after clinical signs have appeared, ending in serious disease or death; and (c) limitation of infection to a single host species and localization of anatomical lesions in a single organ or tissue system.

In this paper we present additional data on the transmissibility and serial passage of scrapie to mice with cell-free filtrates and new filtration data on the size of the virus, confirm its unusual thermostability as compared to most other viruses, report data on the density of scrapie virus as determined by cesium chloride density gradient centrifugation, illustrate our failure to demonstrate immune antibody in naturally or experimentally infected animals, and discuss the probable reasons for failure to demonstrate clearly any antibody in sera from animals hyperimmunized with scrapie-infected sheep or mouse brain suspensions. In addition, we present a summary of our program on attempts to transmit subacute and chronic degenerative diseases of the human central nervous system to a variety of mammalian and avian hosts and, finally, we report the current status of our work on the successful transmission of a Kuru-like syndrome to chimpanzees from brain suspensions of Kuru victims. The preliminary data were summarized recently (GAJDUSEK et al., 1966).

The strain of scrapie virus we have employed in most of our studies is the Compton strain designated SPG 9, isolated by CHANDLER from a sheep in England and subsequently adapted by him to goats. The virus was in the ninth goat passage when received in our laboratory, where it has been easily adapted to several strains of mice. In addition, we have isolated many strains of the scrapie virus in groups of mice inoculated with separate brain specimens of United States sheep naturally infected with scrapie. Although the incubation period of the virus in mice inoculated with sheep tissue may range from 12 to 15 months before clinical disease is observed, the virus adapts easily to mice after several passages and the incubation period is then 4 to 6 months.

Results of Scrapie Studies

The data tabulated in Table 1 illustrate the serial transmissibility of the scrapie virus in mice by the intracerebral or intraperitoneal routes following storage either as frozen or lyophilized stock seed suspensions. Clinically the mice develop hyperexcitability, drowsiness, waddling incoordinated gait, emaciation, a stiff almost catatonic tail, and in many instances, a urinary and fecal incontinence and persistent priapism; the neuropathological lesions consist of marked astrogliosis, vacuolation, loss of neurons and myelin degeneration, predominantly of the cerebellar and hypothalamic systems, and absence of inflammatory lesions. The pathogenesis of the virus in mice as reported by EKLUND et al. (1964) shows a widespread distribution of the virus, first in the reticuloendothelial system and only much later in the central nervous system, the target organ.

Table 1. *Serial propagation of scrapie virus in mice*

Strain designation	Passage level	Age of mice (in days)	Route of inoculation	Infectivity titer ($\log_{10}\mathrm{LD}_{50}$)
SPG9*	M/1	40	i.c.	$10^{-5.6}$
	M/2 (wet)	35	i.c.	$10^{-6.0}$
	M/2 (post lyophilization)	17	i.c.	$10^{-6.0}$
			i.p.	$10^{-6.1}$
	M/3	40	i.c.	$10^{-5.5}$
			i.p.	$10^{-4.7}$
		20	i.c.	$10^{-5.3}$
			i.p.	$10^{-5.2}$
	M/4	30	i.c.	$10^{-8.1}$

* Brain of ninth passage in goats of Compton strain.

Estimate of size by filtration

It was of interest to determine the size of the scrapie virus particle inasmuch as such information in the literature was at best speculative. A 10% suspension of the scrapie infected mouse brain tissue in phosphate buffered physiological saline (pH 7.4) was centrifuged at 5000 rpm for 30 minutes, the supernatant fluid then serially passed through gradacol membranes of 520 mμ, 220 mμ, 82 mμ, 43 mμ, 27 mμ, and 8 mμ diameters. Serial dilutions of filtrates were inoculated intracerebrally into litters of three-to five-day-old Swiss mice. As shown in Table 2, deaths attributable to scrapie occurred with all filtrates through membranes down to and including 43 mμ pore diameter, but particles infectious for mice were not detected in the filtrate that had passed the 27 mμ membrane nor in the filtrate that had passed the 8 mμ membrane. Thus, the virus is very small in the range of 16 to 26 mμ. In support of these results are data, obtained by ALPER et al. for inactivation of scrapie by ionizing radiation. They calculated the "target size" of scrapie to be approximately 7 mμ (1966). While data from these later experiments would place scrapie among the smallest of viruses, the results are based on the size of the infective core rather than the entire virus particle. Nevertheless, the small size of the virus would help to explain some of its unorthodox characteristics, such as resistance to ultraviolet irradiation and to inactivation by organic solvents tested. In collaboration with Dr. PAVEL ALBRECHT of our laboratory, we recently performed a series of experiments to further assay the size of the virus as well as the susceptibility of virus infectivity to ultraviolet irradiation, RNAse and DNAse.

Table 2. *Determination of particle size of scrapie agent by gradacol membrane filtration*

Dilution of inoculum*	Pre-filtration infectivity titer	Ability of selected filtrates to induce scrapie disease in mice**					
		520 mμ filtrate	220 mμ filtrate	82 mμ filtrate	43 mμ filtrate	27 mμ filtrate	8 mμ filtrate
10^{-1}					6/6	0/10	0/10
10^{-2}				6/6	9/9	0/8	
10^{-3}	9/9	6/6	6/6	6/6	5/6		
10^{-4}	11/11	6/6	6/7				
10^{-5}	5/5	2/3	0/2				
10^{-6}	0/7	4/9	0/6				
10^{-7}	0/6	0/6					
10^{-8}	0/2	0/7					
10^{-9}		0/11					
LD_{50}	$10^{-5.5}$	$10^{-5.7}$	$10^{-4.4}$	$>10^{-3.0}$	$>10^{-3.0}$	$<10^{-1.0}$	$<10^{-1.0}$

* Virus was in the form of a 10% mouse brain suspension in isotonic physiological saline-phosphate buffer (pH7.4) clarified by centrifugation at 5,000 rpm/30 minutes.

** Expressed as the number of mice developing scrapie/number of mice inoculated.

Thermostability

Scrapie virus in crude mouse brain is more resistant to thermal inactivation than other "more conventional viruses". This observation, first made by CHANDLER (1961), has been confirmed in our laboratory. Suspensions of scrapie-infected mouse brain tissue were prepared in isotonic phosphate buffered saline, clarified by centrifugation at 2500 rpm for 30 minutes, and aliquots, both undiluted 10% suspensions and suspensions serially diluted tenfold in phosphate buffered saline, were distributed into glass ampules which were then sealed and immersed in a stationary position in mechanically agitated constant temperature (100° C) water for varying time intervals. As may be noted in Table 3, while approximately 4 logs of virus, 99.9% of the infectivity, were destroyed by exposure to 100° C for 15 minutes, such a temperature cannot be relied upon to produce total inactivation. However, it should be noted that in preparations containing less proteinaceous material, the agent might be less heat resistant, although in our experiments done on the virus serially diluted before exposure (see Table 3), the 10^{-2} dilution of infected brain tissue remained infectious after exposure to 100° C for 10 minutes.

Table 3. *Thermostability of scrapie agent following exposure to 100° C temperature for varying periods of time*

Dilution of mouse brain suspension	Treatment										
	Experiment I			Experiment II							
	None	Exposure to 100°C/15 min		Serial dilutions exposed to 100°C (time in min)							
		Diluted before exposure	Diluted after exposure *	None	2	5	10	15	30	45	60
10^{-1}	10/10 **	5/8	4/5	5/6		0/3	0/3	0/5	0/4	0/4	0/7
10^{-2}	10/10	3/6	1/5	6/6	2/4	0/6	0/3	0/2	0/4	0/4	0/4
10^{-3}	10/10	0/7	1/8	6/6	0/5	0/3	3/7	0/5	0/5	0/5	0/5
10^{-4}	3/3	0/10	1/6	3/3	0/5	0/3	0/4	0/6	0/6	0/5	0/4
10^{-5}	7/8	0/5	0/6	2/3	0/4	0/7	0/4	0/6	0/5	0/4	0/4
10^{-6}	0/9	0/8	0/6	0/5	1/5	0/2	0/2	0/6	0/5	0/5	
10^{-7}	0/10	0/8	0/8	0/7	0/7	0/3					
10^{-8}	0/10	0/8	0/8	0/4	1/3	0/3					
LD_{50}	$10^{-5.4}$	$10^{-1.6}$	$10^{-1.6}$	$10^{-5.0}$	$10^{-2.0}$	$<10^{-1.0}$	$\sim10^{-2.0}$	$<10^{-1.0}$	$<10^{-1.0}$	$<10^{-1.0}$	$<10^{-1.0}$

* Exposed as a 10^{-1} dilution.

** Mortality ratio = number of mice developing scrapie/number of mice inoculated; Experiment I held for 750 days post inoculation; Experiment II summarized 560 days post inoculation.

Table 4. *Infectivity and density gradient of scrapie virus in cesium chloride*

Virus	Dilutions of inoculum	Scrapie disease in mice (no. of animals dead/no. of animals inoculated)						
		10,000 rpm 30 min	10,000 rpm/30 min supernatant fluid layered in saturated cesium chloride and centrifuged 39,000 rpm/24 hours					
			Fraction 1–1 1.413	Fraction 1–2 1.392	Fraction 1–3 1.370	Fraction 1–4 1.319	Fraction 1–5 1.292	Fraction 1–6 1.259
Scrapie	10^{-2}	10/10	2/4	2/4		5/5	2/5	4/4
infected	10^{-3}	11/11	0/5	0/6	4/4	6/6	4/4	0/5
mouse	10^{-4}	11/11	0/4	0/5	4/6	4/5	2/5	0/6
brain sus-	10^{-5}	11/11	0/4	0/5	0/5	0/4	0/4	0/6
pension	10^{-6}	0/6	0/4	0/3	0/5	0/4	0/4	0/6
SPG 9:	10^{-7}	0/5	0/4	0/4	0/5	0/4	0/5	0/6
M 4	10^{-8}	0/5	0/6	0/4	0/4	0/6	0/5	0/6
Mouse IC LD$_{50}$/0.02 ml:		$10^{-5.5}$	$10^{-2.0}$	$10^{-2.0}$	$10^{-4.2}$	$10^{-4.4}$	$10^{-3.4}$	$10^{-2.5}$

Table 5. *Attempts to demonstrate neutralizing antibody to mouse scrapie agent*

Virus dilution	Scrapie agent mixed with *:									
	Sheep serum[a]		Mouse serum[a]		Mouse immune ascitic fluid[b]		Rooster serum[b]		Rabbit serum[b]	
	Normal	Scrapie	Normal	Scrapie	Normal	Scrapie	Normal	Scrapie	Normal	Scrapie
10^{-1}	6/6**	8/8	10/10	8/8	5/5	5/5	5/5	5/5	5/5	5/5
10^{-2}	8/8	8/8	10/10	8/8	5/5	5/5	5/5	5/5	5/5	5/5
10^{-3}	7/7	8/8	10/10	8/8	5/5	5/5	5/5	5/5	5/5	5/5
10^{-4}	8/8	8/8	3/3	4/4	5/5	5/5	5/5	5/5	5/5	5/5
10^{-5}	8/8	7/8	7/8	6/7	5/5	5/5	5/5	5/5	5/5	5/5
10^{-6}	2/9	0/5	0/9	0/7	5/5	5/5	5/5	5/5	5/5	5/5
10^{-7}	0/9	0/8	0/10	0/5	5/5	5/5	5/5	5/5	5/5	5/5
10^{-8}	0/9	0/8	0/10							
$MICLD_{50}$	$10^{-5.6}$	$10^{-5.4}$	$10^{-5.4}$	$10^{-5.4}$	$\geqq 10^{-7.5}$	$\geqq 10^{-7.5}$	$\geqq 10^{-7.5}$	$\geqq 10^{-7.5}$	$\geqq 10^{-7.5}$	$\geqq 10^{-7.5}$

* Mixture of undiluted serum, or ascitic fluid (inactivaded 56° C/30 min) and 10-fold dilutions of mouse brain infected with scrapie virus: [a] Serum-virus mixtures incubated at 37° C for 1 hour, then inoculated into 6–8 gm mice by the intracerebral route. [b] Serum-virus mixtures incubated at room temperature (25°–27° C) for 16–18 hours, then inoculated into litters of 5- to 7-day-old mice by the intracerebral route.

** Number of mice developing scrapie/number of mice inoculated.

HUNTER (1965) has recently reported that the critical temperature for rapid heat inactivation of scrapie virus is 87.5° C; at lower temperatures the inactivation is extremely slow.

Cesium chloride density gradient studies

In order to characterize scrapie virus by physicochemical methods, an attempt was made to determine the density of the virus in our density gradient centrifugation using cesium chloride gradient with centrifugation at 39,000 rpm for 24 hours. The infectivity for mice injected intracerebrally with the different fractions and the corresponding density is illustrated in Table 4. Maximum virus concentration was detected in that fraction whose density was about 1.32. This suggests that the virus is not dense enough to be a naked nucleic acid, as some people have hypothesized, but, on the other hand, too dense to contain a lipid coat. It was feasible to precipitate non-viral protein with fluorocarbon but considerable loss of infectivity was observed after vigorous two-fold treatment with Gentron-112.

Failure to demonstrate antibody to scrapie virus

The most disturbing aspect of the study of scrapie has surely been the consistent failure to demonstrate antibody to the virus by any of the many techniques that have been employed. Complement fixation, precipitation, gel-diffusion, direct and indirect fluorescent antibody techniques have been unsuccessful to date. Neutralization attempts by numerous modifications of the conventional virus neutraliza-

Table 6. *Attempts to demonstrate neutralizing antibody to scrapie*

| Serum incubation: | 37° C/l hr. | | 4° C/24 hrs. | | 27° C/72 hrs. |
inoculation:	IP	SC	IP	SC	IC
Pre-rabbit 131	5.5	4.3	5.3	4.0	4.6
Post rabbit 131	4.8	3.8	4.7	3.4	4.5
Post rabbit 111	ND	ND	4.7	3.4	4.8
Post rooster 46	ND	ND	3.8	3.6	ND
Human 1595	ND	ND	6.0	ND	5.0
None	4.8	4.0	4.8	3.8	5.0

tion test as shown in Tables 5 and 6 failed to demonstrate presence of antiviral antibody. Furthermore, the data presented in Table 7 show that passive protection type tests, such as those required to demonstrate neutralization of hog cholera virus, by inoculating serum into test animals two to four hours before the virus dilutions are injected peripherally, have yielded questionably significant neutralization indices. Sera from both normal and scrapie affected sheep and mice and also sera of monkeys, roosters and rabbits immunized by repeated injections of scrapie infected mouse brain suspensions have been used in these neutralization tests.

Unless the concentration of antigen in infected mouse brain tissue (LD$_{50}$ titer 10^{-6}) is too low to provoke an antibody response, some other mechanism has to be

4*

postulated in order to explain the inability of scrapie to evoke an immune response demonstrable by the currently available techniques.

Thus, although most investigators now agree that the etiologic agent of scrapie is a virus, many biological and physical properties require better and more detailed

Table 7. *Mouse passive protection type neutralization test with scrapie*

Serum	Dilution of serum	Virus titer ($\log_{10}LD_{50}/.3\,ml\,SC$)	Neutralization index
Normal monkey	1:10	4.4	
Post monkey 604-0	1:10	3.9	0.5
Post monkey 622-N	1:10	4.0	0.4
Post monkey 637-N	1:10	4.5	
Post monkey 643-N	1:10	4.7	
Pre-rabbit 13130	1:5	4.5	
Post 128 days	1:5	4.8	
Post 342 days	1:5	3.6	0.9
Post 483 days	1:5	3.7	0.8
Normal sheep undiluted		5.6	
Scrapie terminal sheep 103529 E undiluted		5.4	
Pre-rooster 84 E	1:8	4.6	
Post 60 days	1:8	4.7	

definition before the true nature of the virus is clearly understood. Nevertheless, it continues to aid in the gathering of data directly applicable to our study of human diseases.

Results of Kuru Studies

In 1964 (GAJDUSEK and GIBBS) and 1965 (GIBBS and GAJDUSEK), we described in detail our program of work on the possible infectious etiology of subacute and chronic human central nervous system diseases. We presented negative results on isolation and experimental transmission following 19 and 21 months of observation of a variety of several species of many different hosts. These included chimpanzees, monkeys, and smaller animals inoculated with suspensions of human brain and other tissues obtained at surgical biopsy or early autopsy and preserved under optimal conditions of liquid nitrogen or mechanically controlled temperatures of lower than —70° C. The diseases under study included Kuru, amyotrophic lateral sclerosis, Parkinson's disease, amyotrophic lateral sclerosis-Parkinsonism dementia syndrome observed in Chamorro natives of Guam, subacute inclusion body encephalitis, multiple sclerosis, Schilder's disease, progressive multifocal leukoencephalopathy and necrotizing encephalitis.

In early 1966 (GAJDUSEK et al.) we presented details of the apparent transmission of Kuru to chimpanzees and of our present efforts at virus isolation from tissues from these animals and from Kuru patients. A clinical syndrome, resem-

Table 8. *Results of attempts to transmit kuru to chimpanzees*

Patient	Primary isolation studies						Second passage		Reisolation	
	Chimpanzee	Date of inoculation	Onset of disease	Incubation period (months)	Date of sacrifice or death	Course of illness (months)	Chimpanzee	Date of inoculation	Chimpanzee	Date of inoculation
I Eiro	Georgette	Sep. 63	May 65	20	Oct. 65	5	Herman	Oct. 65		
							Billey	Oct. 65		
							Susy	Oct. 65		
									Henry	Oct. 65
									Freddie	Oct. 65
									Snappy	Oct. 65
							Connie	Mar. 66		
							Ringo	Mar. 66		
							Elvis	Mar. 66		
							23	Mar. 66		
							Lena	Mar. 66		
II Kigea	Daisey	Aug. 63	May 65	21	Feb. 66	9				
III Kabuinampa	Joanne	Feb. 64	Aug. 65	18	Apr. 66	8				
IV Kariwani	Happy	Nov. 63	Dec. 65	25	May 66	6				
	Joker	Nov. 63	Apr. 66	29	Jun. 66	3				
V Enage	Zeke	Aug. 63	Feb. 66	30	May 66	4				
VI Moba	Charlene	Sep. 63	Feb. 66	29	May 66	4				
VII Igierakaba	Oscar	Feb. 64								
VIII Kwase	Moe	Apr. 66								
	Joe	Apr. 66								

bling Kuru in man, has now developed in seven of the eight chimpanzees 18 to 30 months after intracerebral inoculation with brain suspension from different Kuru patients. This fatal syndrome with progressive cerebellar ataxia and incoordination has not been seen as a spontaneous disease of apes and is the most encouraging evidence to date of the transmissibility of one of the subacute or chronic human central nervous system diseases under investigation in our program.

Results of the experiments in chimpanzees are summarized in Table 8. It is noteworthy that the incubation period in the seven affected animals has ranged from 18 to 30 months. The interval between the appearance of the first clinical signs and the sacrifice of the animals was 5 and 9 months, respectively, for the chimpanzee No. 4 – Georgette and chimpanzee No. 1 – Daisy, while the third chimpanzee No. 9 – Joanne died after eight months of illness. Most remarkable, however, is the close similarity in the clinical appearance of the syndrome in the chimpanzees to Kuru in human patients. To document and preserve this clinical record, "research cinema" film techniques were used extensively, and several research films are in preparation illustrating the progress of the disease in chimpanzees.

For the purpose of this presentation, we will give a brief description of the disease of chimpanzee No. 4, Georgette, to illustrate the typical syndrome observed in these animals. Chimpanzee No. 4, a female of about 2 years of age, was inoculated intracerebrally in September, 1963 with 0.2 ml of a 10% brain suspension obtained from Eiro (Eiru) a boy of Fore of age 13, had died in September, 1962 (Tables 8 and 9). Brain material of this patient, frozen within 4.5 hours of death, was kept in a refrigerator (–10° C) or in dry ice until placed in storage at –70° C 60 hours after death. In May, 1965, chimpanzee No. 4 first showed signs of apathy and lassitude, which progressed and within a month were accompanied by a pendulous lower lip, increased sensitivity to cold, and piloerection. Within two months she demonstrated titubation and trunkal unsteadiness, a wide-based, lurching gait, and later, marked dipmetria of hand movements. Her ataxia became more severe and she suffered many stumbles and falls. Eventually she was unable to sit up without external support and spent her time huddled at the bottom of her cage. She required encouragement to eat and drink, but only terminally was there any difficulty with swallowing. Visual fixation became impaired terminally. Hearing appeared normal. There was no spontaneous nystagmus, but it could be elicited by vestibular stimulation. At no time was there any motor paresis, though power was poorly sustained; passive limb tone was normal or decreased. There was no loss of pain sensation; hyperaesthesia to touch occurred over the last 6 weeks of her illness. Detectable reflex changes, changes in the fundi, convulsion, impairment of consciousness or obvious disorientation did not occur. Hematological, biochemical, and trace metal determinations on the blood were considered normal. Cerebrospinal fluid collected just before death was clear with a protein level of 237 mg/100 ml. Progressive ataxia involving the trunk and all limbs and leading to increased disability remained the chief feature of the syndrome. This animal as well as the second animal was killed when her terminal debility, dysphagia and respiratory distress caused our concern lest sudden death from secondary infection should intervene.

There were no gross neuropathological lesions other than a fine needle scar at the site of the inoculation in the frontal lobe. Preliminary histological study, by Mrs. E. BECK and Professor P. M. DANIELS, of the Maudsley Institute in London, England, revealed the diffuse non-specific changes seen in the brains of Kuru victims such as generalized astrocytic hypertrophy and widespread status spongiosus together with the more selective degenerations seen in the cerebellum.

Table 9. *Kuru in chimpanzees*

Patient	Primary inoculation	Incubation period (months)	Duration (months)	Second passage	Inoculum
I	Sept. 63	20	5	Oct. 65	10^{-1}
				Oct. 65	10^{-1}
				Oct. 65	10^{-1}
				Mar. 66	10^{-3}
				Mar. 66	10^{-5}
				Mar. 66	10^{-1} 220 mμ filtrate
				Mar. 66	10^{-1} 100 mμ filtrate
				Mar. 66	10^{-1} ip+sc
	Oct. 65				
	Oct. 65				
	Oct. 65				
II	Aug. 63	21	9		
III	Feb. 64	18	8		
IV	Nov. 63	25	6		
	Nov. 63	29	3		
V	Aug. 63	30	4		
VI	Sept. 63	29	4		
VII	Feb. 64				
VIII	Apr. 66				
	Apr. 66				

When this first affected chimpanzee was killed on the 163rd day of illness, generous portions of blood, brain and visceral tissue were taken and stored in liquid nitrogen, using separate sterile instruments for each tissue. In addition, a freshly prepared 10% suspension of unfrozen brain material, pooled from three brain areas, was inoculated intracerebrally into three young chimpanzees and a number of individual monkeys of several species. As noted in Table 9, we have inoculated chimpanzees and several species of monkeys intracerebrally with 10^{-3} and 10^{-5} dilutions of the chimpanzee brain suspension, other chimpanzees and monkeys with 220 mμ filtrates and 100 mμ filtrates; and a single chimpanzee was inoculated peripherally only. Three young chimpanzees were also inoculated intracerebrally with the original 10% Eiro brain suspension. Additional chimpanzees were injected intracerebrally and peripherally with visceral tissue suspensions prepared from human Kuru victims, from chimpanzees that have died with Kuru-like syndrome, with undiluted serum from humans whose CNS tissues in suspension have induced the disease in chimpanzees, and sera from other human Kuru victims. Further, just recently brain tissue specimens in suspension from the two human Kuru patients (Eiro and Kigea), brain tissue suspensions from chimpanzee No. 4 and chimpanzee No. 1, brain tissue from a human with amyotrophic lateral sclerosis, and brain tissue from a child with subacute inclusion body encephalitis were individually inoculated into various species of animals listed in Table 10.

Attempts are made to isolate an agent from these tissues in a variety of tissue culture systems, in chick embryos and in 17 genetically defined strains of mice (Table 10) as well as in other small laboratory animals. Explants of the central nervous system tissue and visceral organs of the chimpanzees are being closely studied for unusual morphological lesions compared to normal tissue explants, and for resistance to superinfection with other viruses such as the adenoviruses and for isolation studies by inoculation of fluids from these explants into established cell lines. Finally, animals that have not developed clinical disease during the many months of observation following inoculation are treated with immuno-suppressant drugs and subjected to other forms of treatment which may activate latent agents. It is strongly suspected, however, that presence of homologous antibodies *in vivo* does not play a significant role in determining the incubation period nor the course of the disease.

Table 10. *Summary of experimental hosts used in inoculation program*

Primates	Other mammals	Avian

Chimpanzees	Sheep
	  Cheviot
	  Suffolk
		Turkeys
		  Noryork

Rhesus
  Newborn
  Immatures
	Pigs
	  Chester whites
	  Dorchester
		Ducks
		  Long Island

Cynomolgus
  Newborn
  Immatures
	Goats
	  Mixed breeds
		Geese
		  Domestic

African green (aethiops)
  Immatures
Slow loris
	Hamsters
	  Golden Syrian
		Chickens
		  White leghorns
		  Embryonated eggs
		  Day old chicks

Barbary apes (S· sylvania)
  Immatures
	Guinea pigs
	  Hartley strain	

Spider	Mice 17 genetically defined	
Squirrel	lines	

In view of the close similarity in the clinical picture and the wide neuropathological findings of Kuru in man with those of scrapie in sheep and mice, the remote possibility of scrapie infection in the affected chimpanzees must be considered.

Thus far there is no evidence of the scrapie virus producing disease in primates. All primates inoculated with human material are housed in a remote building separate from that in which scrapie investigations are being carried out. Of 57 chimpanzees and more than 300 smaller monkeys in these transmission experiments from human tissue, no animals have developed a chronic progressive neurological disorder, other than the seven Kuru-inoculated chimpanzees described herein. Rhesus monkeys inoculated 23 months ago with scrapie mouse brain suspension have not yet shown disease. Two chimpanzees have been inoculated intracerebrally and intraperitoneally, respectively, with scrapie material as have additional species of monkeys; however, because of the difficulty in obtaining chimpanzees, these experiments were initiated only four months ago.

There is a remarkable similarity between the course and clinical syndrome of Kuru in man and the clinical syndrome induced experimentally in the chimpanzee. The fact that the experimental disease was observed in seven of eight chimpanzees inoculated, in all but one instance with brain material from a different Kuru patient, that the onset occurred after a similar long incubation period in each chimpanzee, that the neuropathological findings in the experimental disease in the cases thus far examined resemble those observed in Kuru victims, and that there is no recorded case of such disease in non-inoculated chimpanzees lead us to conclude that Kuru has been transmitted experimentally to these chimpanzees.

References

Two monographs have recently appeared that summarize much of the work by ourselves and others on the viruses and diseases discussed in this paper:

a) Report of Scrapie Seminar, ARS 91—55, Agricultural Research Service, U. S. Department of Agriculture, January 27—30, 1964.

b) Slow, Latent and Temporate Virus Infections, D. C. GAJDUSEK, C. J. GIBBS, JR., and M. ALPERS (ed.), NINDB Monograph No. 2, PHS No. 1378. Washington; U. S. Government Printing Office, 1965.

ALPER, T., D. A. HAIG, and M. C. CLARKE: The exceptionally small size of the scrapie agent. Biochem. biophys. Res. Commun. 22, 278—283 (1966).

CHANDLER, R. L.: Encephalopathy in mice produced with scrapie brain material. Lancet I, 1378—1379, 1961.

EKLUND, C. M., R. C. KENNEDY, and W. J. HADLOW: Evolution of scrapie virus infection in mice. Report of scrapie seminar, ARS 91—53, p. 288—291, Agricultural Research Service, U. S. Department of Agriculture, January 27—30, 1964.

GAJDUSEK, D. C.: Kuru. Trans. roy. Soc. trop. Med. Hyg. 57, 151—159 (1963).

—, and C. J. GIBBS, JR.: Attempts to demonstrate a transmissible agent in Kuru, amyotrophic lateral sclerosis, and other subacute and chronic nervous system degenerations of man. Nature (Lond.) 204, 257—259 (1964).

— —, and M. ALPERS: Experimental transmission of a Kuru-like syndrome to chimpanzees. Nature (Lond.) 209, 794—796 (1966).

—, and V. ZIGAS: Degenerative disease of the central nervous system in New Guinea. The endemic occurrence of Kuru in the native population. New Engl. J. Med. 267, 974—978 (1957).

GIBBS, JR., C. J., and D. C. GAJDUSEK: Attempts to demonstrate a transmissible agent in Kuru, amyotrophic lateral sclerosis, and other sub-acute chronic progressive nervous system degenerations of man, p. 39—48. In: D. C. GAJDUSEK, C. J. GIBBS, JR., and

M. Alpers (ed.), NINDB Monograph No. 2, Slow, Latent and Temperate Virus Infections, PHS No 1378. Washington; U. S. Government Printing Office 1965.

Gordon, W. S.: Advances in veterinary sciences. Vet. Rec. 58, 516—520 (1946).

Hunter, G. D., and G. C. Millison: Studies on the heat stability and chromatographic behavior of the scrapie agent. J. gen. Microbiol. 37, 251—258 (1964).

Palsson, P. A., I. H. Pattison, and E. J. Field: Transmission experiments with multiple sclerosis p. 49—54. In: D. C. Gajdusek, C. J. Gibbs Jr., and M. Alpers (ed.), NINDB Monograph No. 2, Slow, Latent, and Temperate Virus Infections, PHS No. 1378. Washington: U. S. Government Printing Office, 1965.

Sigurdsson, B.: Observations on three slow infections of sheep. Brit. vet. J. 110, 255—270, 307—322, 341—354 (1954).

Stamp, J. T.: Scrapie disease of sheep. A review of the contradictory evidence as to the nature of the disease. Vet. Rec. 70, 50—55 (1958).

Zilber, L. A., Z. L. Baidakova, A. M. Gardashian, N. V. Konovalov, T. L. Bunina, and E. M. Barabadze: Possible viral etiology of amyotrophic lateral sclerosis. Vop. Virus. 5, 520—528 (1962).

Discussion on Kuru, Scrapie and the Experimental Kuru-Like Syndrome in Chimpanzees

CARLETON GAJDUSEK

National Institute of Neurological Diseases and Blindness,
National Institutes of Health, Bethesda, Md.

It is strangely interesting that scrapie, a degenerative disease of the central nervous system of sheep, and kuru, a rare degenerative disease of the central nervous system of man in the Eastern Highlands of New Guinea and restricted to the Fore peoples and their immediate neighbors, have given rise to a large portion of world research activity in the field of slow virus infections. Dr. GIBBS has reviewed the quest for infectious agents in chronic and subacute degenerative diseases of the central nervous system which has been in progress in our laboratories for the past several years, with particular attention to scrapie, the infection on which Dr. MORRIS, Dr. GIBBS, and I began to work after HADLOW had brought to my attention the remarkable similarities in the neuropathology and course between kuru in man and scrapie in sheep (HADLOW, 1959). Dr. GIBBS has also brought our previous report of transmission of a kuru-like disease to chimpanzees (GAJDUSEK *et al.*, 1966) up to date with the final score of seven cases of kuru-like syndrome in eight chimpanzees inoculated with human kuru brain material. It is this first successful transmission of a subacute or chronic central nervous system degeneration of man to primate that has excited our imagination and raised our hopes that other subacute and chronic degenerative nervous system disorders may also be transmissible.

However, it remains to be emphasized that although we believe we have transmitted kuru to chimpanzees, we have not yet proved that it is serially transmissible, that the agent is filterable and, thus, possibly a virus, nor have we by any means fulfilled all of KOCH's postulates. Thus, the crude 10% human brain suspension with which we started has not been filtered, and could contain bacteria, fungi or protozoa, mycoplasmas, rickettsias, spirochetes, leptospiras or other microorganisms larger than viruses. The failure to detect any of these by *in vitro* culture, by injection of chick embryos and other animals, including other primates, and the failure to demonstrate either such microorganisms in histopathology, or even an inflammatory reaction in the brain with perivascular cuffing, has prompted us to suspect that the agent is filterable. The experiments to establish that it is serially transmissible, filterable, and finally, to determine its size by filtration — assuming that it is serially transmissible — we have only recently initiated. Furthermore, the same six inocula which caused the kuru-like syndrome in our seven chimpanzees after a delay of 18 to 30 months has failed to cause any illness in smaller laboratory animals, including many other species of monkeys held under observation for an even longer period of time. Thus, we already have clear-cut evidence for marked genetic or species specificity of susceptibility to the disease.

Whether we have here the first slow virus infection of man transmitted to a laboratory animal and a fine experimental model for natural kuru, or some previously unreported spontaneous disease of primates, a previously unknown type of experimental allergic encephalomyelitis (only 0.2 ml of 10% brain suspension has been inoculated intracerebrally, and control animals with non-kuru brain inocula remain normal thus far), a most unlikely but frightening contamination of our animals with scrapie virus which to date is not known to cause disease in primates, or some exotic viral-enzyme interaction, remains to be proved.

Pathologically, the brains of the kuru chimpanzees show most of the changes associated with kuru in man (Beck et al., 1966) but these are overridden by an intensive status spongiosus (Albrecht, 1966; Beck, 1966; Klatzo, 1966). Status spongiosus is found in the brains of human kuru patients, but it appears so severely in the chimpanzee brains as to command attention and invite speculation on the problem of its pathogenesis. The work of Bignami and Palladini (1966), brought to my attention by Mrs. Beck, gives a metabolic model of enzyme inhibition-induced pathology akin to the status spongiosus seen in human kuru, in experimentally transmitted scrapie, in naturally occurring mink encephalopathy, and in our kuru-like syndrome in chimpanzees. These investigators produced a devastating status spongiosus in the brains of rats by application of ouabain, a specific inhibitor of the membrane ATPase enzyme system controlling cell membrane permeability to Na^+ and K^+ ions in brain cells. With this model in mind, one is temped to add to the dozens of facile theoretical formulations about kuru and scrapie: Can a slow virus agent progressively deplete the supply, or interfere with the action, of an enzyme to produce, thereby, a reduction of membrane ATPase activity to a critical level? This would be expressed, as in ouabain-induced enzyme block, by a spongiform degeneration in the brain. Species and breeds or races, or even individuals, with different levels of such an enzyme might, in such a case, be differently vulnerable to the damaging effects of slow virus proliferation in their brain cells. There are well understood mechanisms in molecular genetics to account for such differences in enzyme activity by heterozygous-homozygous gene dosage effects, or by pleomorphisms in the enzyme synthesis coding loci resulting in enzyme varieties of differing activities. Unlike most of the other theories which have been cluttering the literature with speculations on kuru and scrapie, this rather wild one, for which I, as a gamesman, would hold little hope, at least suggests some specific experiments and testing measurements that are not already underway before it is advanced, and thus it has some small zustification for being stated. We shall be looking experimentally at this rather far-fetched possibility.

The transmission of kuru experimentally leaves no suggestion that passage of the scrapie virus or of some other contaminating agent or a spontaneous disease of chimpanzees has occurred, because the many control chimpanzees in the laboratory remain well, and the seven brain inocula have been obtained at different times from six different kuru patients. However, it must be noted that our laboratory reporting this work is deeply involved in scrapie investigation. The recent report of multiple sclerosis brain inducing scrapie in sheep in one laboratory (PÁLSSON *et al.*, 1965), and not in another (DICK *et al.*, 1965) point to the cause for concern. On the other hand, the scrapie agent is not known to induce disease in primates. High-titrating scrapie infected mouse brain suspensions have, after three years, caused no disease in rhesus and cynomologus monkeys (HADLOW, 1966, and our own data); but chimpanzees inoculated with scrapie have only been observed for five months and not yet for periods comparable to the incubation periods in experimental kuru. No spontaneous disease of chimpanzees suggesting a kuru-like syndrome has been reported.

Although scrapie is easily transmitted from infected sheep to other sheep, goats, mice, rats and hamsters, nevertheless, even to direct intracerebral challenge, there is a markedly different resistance to disease between different breeds of sheep and between sheep and goats. Further, although contact and oral route infection with the scrapie virus has been established in the laboratory, the irregular epidemiological pattern seen in natural sheep scrapie remains without explanation. Further investigation is needed to determine whether genetic susceptibility to a very widespread agent or some more subtle genetic mechanisms are involved in the epidemiology of natural scrapie in sheep.

Similarly, the failure to observe a single instance of kuru through contact in non-Fore-related persons, in spite of their long residence in the kuru region, and the strange recent disappearance of cases among younger children (ALPERS and GAJDUSEK, 1966) suggest as yet unsuspected peculiarities in the mechanisms of transmission and pathogenesis in the natural disease. We have wondered whether cannibalism with the consumption of their deceased relatives, which was until recently prevalent among the Fore, served to introduce to the people and spread through their population a slow virus to which they may be more genetically susceptible than are their neighbors, or served in some way to sensitize them to, or activate, a rather ubiquitous latent viral agent. Earlier, we wondered whether hypersensitivity to brain tissue might not have been established by the consumption in early childhood of brain tissue from deceased relatives, even of those dying of kuru. None of the hypotheses finds support from our field epidemiological work or search in kuru tissues for evidence of autoimmune reaction.

The scrapie agent is for several reasons bizarre and disturbingly different among viruses. It possesses unusual thermostability and resistance to formaldehyde, to enzymes, and to other chemical agents, and to pH for a virus. Very small particle size, as estimated by some of the conflicting data on filtration, and the difficulty thus far in producing a detectable antibody to the scrapie agent, further add to the confusion. Recent data by ALPER, HAIG and CLARKE (1966) on the exceptionally small size of the agent as determined by calculation of target size from radiation inactivation in a high energy electron beam, and their failure to inactivate the agent by high energy dosage of ultraviolet radiation, add further chapters to the scrapie fairy tale. If these remarkable observations can be substantiated, it will be difficult to maintain our current conviction that in scrapie we are dealing with a conventional virus particle. More likely, it contains a rather small nucleic acid moiety (6–7 mμ), enclosed in rather stable protein capsid of small virus diameter (15–20 mμ diameter) and it may well belong to the group of defective viruses as do the Rous sarcoma virus associated agents and adenovirus associated agents. Failure thus far of all *in vitro* immunological systems to detect the agent may well rest on the failure to obtain adequate virus titers in immunizing antigen preparations and similar failure with the reagent antigens used in the tests.

Finally, the most satisfactory interpretation of the kuru-like syndrome now seen in seven chimpanzees each inoculated with one of six different kuru brain suspensions is that kuru disease itself has been transmitted to the chimpanzees. The remote possibility that scrapie has been inadvertently introduced in such a remarkable pattern into the chimpanzee colony would lead to the perhaps more disturbing possibility that the scrapie agent could produce the devastating degeneration of kuru in the chimpanzee — presumably also in man. Furthermore, although the major aim of our virus work is directed toward finding a rapidly replicating system in cell cultures, such as we behold enviously in the hands of Thormar and his colleagues with visna and maedi, it must be remembered that the fascinating features of slow infections of the nervous system are their slowness, their long incubation periods, their long persistent viremias (visna) or high titers of virus in visceral tissues (scrapie), and the remarkable pathological features they induce in the central nervous system (generalized gliosis, demyelination, amyloid plaque formation, status spongiosus, etc.) and the apparently genetic patterns of occurrence of the natural diseases (scrapie and kuru). The chimpanzee model for kuru and the mouse model for scrapie will thus remain important, even when a more readily available cell culture system for studying the agents becomes available.

References

Albrecht, P.: Personal communication (1966).

Alper, T., D. A. Haig and M. C. Clarke: The exceptionally small size of the scrapie agent. Biochem. biophys. Res. Commun. **22**, 278 (1966).

Alpers, M., and D. C. Gajdusek: Changing patterns of kuru: epidemiological changes in the period of increasing contact of the Fore people with western civilization. Amer. J. trop. Med. Hyg. **14**, 852 (1965).

Beck, Elisabeth: Personal communication (1966).

— P. M. Daniel, D. C. Gajdusek, C. J. Gibbs Jr., and M. Alpers: "Experimental kuru" in chimpanzees; a pathological report. Lancet 1966 II, 1056.

Bignami, A., and G. Palladini: Experimentally produced cerebral status spongiosus and continuous pseudorhythmic electro-encephalographic discharges with a membrane-ATPase inhibitor in the rat. Nature (Lond.) **209**, 413 (1966).

Dick, G., J. L. McAlister, Florence McKeowan, and A. M. G. Campbell: Multiple sclerosis and scrapie. J. Neurol. Neurosurg. Psychiat. **28**, 560 (1965).

Gajdusek, D. C., C. J. Gibbs Jr., and M. Alpers: Experimental transmission of a kuru-like syndrome to chimpanzees. Nature (Lond.) **209**, 794 (1966).

— — — Transmission and passage of experimental kuru to chimpanzees. Science, (January), 1967. (In press.)

Hadlow, W. J.: Scrapie and kuru. Lancet 1959 II, 289.

— Personal communications (1966).

KLATZO, I.: Personal communication (1966).
MORRIS, J. A., and D. C. GAJDUSEK: Encephalopathy in mice following inoculation of scrapie sheep brain. Nature (Lond.) **197**, 4872 (1963).
PÁLSSON, P. A., I. H. PATTISON, and E. J. FIELD: Transmission experiments with multiple sclerosis. In: NINDB Monograph No. 2, Slow, Latent and Temperate Virus Infections (GAJDUSEK, GIBBS, and ALPERS, eds.). National Institutes of Health, 49. Washington: U. S. Government Printing Office, 1965.
THORMAR, H.: Paper in this Symposium (1966).

Addendum

Transmission of the kuru syndrome from chimpanzee to chimpanzee has now been effected with a shortening of the incubation period to one year from the 18 to 30 months found on intracerebral passage of human brain tissue to chimpanzees. This intracerebral passage from chimpanzee to chimpanzee hopefully anticipates success in the chimpanzee experiments under way to determine the size and heat stability of the agent, its presence outside of the nervous system, and its pathogenicity by other routes of inoculation.

Concluding Remarks

Symposium on CHINA Viruses

Jacob A. Brody

Epedemiology Branch,
National Institute of Neurological Diseases and Blindness
National Institutes of Health
Bethesda, Maryland

The concept that viruses can cause chronic disease particularly of the nervous system is not a new one (Gajdusek, 1965). Medical literature is rich with suggestions that multiple sclerosis, neuromyelitis optica, and various forms of diffuse cerebral sclerosis are viral diseases. Leukodystrophies and subacute encephalitides are prime candidates for having viral etiologies, particularly when inclusion bodies are prominent. Virus-like particles have been observed by electron microscopy in several instances. There is speculation that diseases such as amyotrophic lateral sclerosis, peroneal muscular atrophy, myasthenia gravis, the presenile dementias of Alzheimer's and Pick's and other central nervous system degenerations may be viral. The remarkable concentration on Guam of amyotrophic lateral sclerosis and Parkinsonism-dementia also suggests viral etiologies (Reed et al., 1966).

On at least four occasions in recent years, Soviet virologists have claimed virus isolations from people with chronic neurologic diseases (Brody et al., 1965). Shubladze reported isolations of a rabies-like virus from multiple sclerosis patients; Zilber described the passage of an agent from amyotrophic lateral sclerosis patients into Rhesus monkeys; Chumakov reported a recovery of the virus of tick-borne encephalitis from a patient with Kozhevnikov's epilepsy (epilepsia partialis continua); and a virus was supposedly isolated from patients with Vilyuisk encephalomyelitis, a strange degenerative disease with progressive pan-encephalitis which is apparently confined to the Yakut people in the area of Vilyuisk in northeastern Siberia. Although none of these virus isolations have been substantiated, they illustrate the approach on the part of Soviet scientists to seek a viral etiology of chronic degenerative diseases of the central nervous system.

The interest and excitement in slow viruses follows years of painstaking work in Iceland with visna, maedi and rida (scrapie), and in England with scrapie (Gajdusek, 1965). We have come now to an important landmark with the probable passage of an infectious agent from humans with kuru into chimpanzees referred to by Dr. Gibbs. This appears to be the best documented association of a virus with a chronic degenerative neurologic disease of humans.

Various types of chronic virus infections are known. There are the latent infections in which the virus is not actively circulating in the host and cannot be demonstrated in his tissues but is present in an altered form and under certain situations becomes manifest. The classic example of this is herpes simplex virus. There are viruses which infect and are present in the circulation or tissues for a long period of time and do not produce detectable pathology, such as adenoviruses in pharyngeal tissue, rat virus in adult rats, or the lactic dehydrogenase (LDH) virus of mice. Some agents cause chronic infection because of unusual immunological situations such as the primary immune tolerance to lymphocoriomeningitis viruses in mice. Another group are agents which are present in the host for long periods of time and eventually produce illness. In some instances disease develops rapidly after a prolonged incubation period such as in rabies or serum hepatitis. In other instances such as in scrapie, visna, and possibly kuru, the illness evolves more slowly and better conforms with our concept of China viruses.

Dr. Johnson in his presentation advanced a very challenging concept of the pathogenesis of some of the slow viruses. The pathology in scrapie, mink encephalitis and kuru differs from that generally associated with virus encephalitis because of the absence of an inflammatory response; nor does it resemble classic autoimmune disease of the central nervous system because primary demyelinization is an inconspicuous feature. What, then, is the virus doing in the nervous tissue and how does it ultimately destroy the cell? Dr. Johnson gave evidence that in infections with rabies, rubella, and mumps the virus could be detected in the cells by immunofluorescent microscopy but by routine pathological techniques the cells were completely normal in appearance. When examined by the electron microscope these cells were loaded with viral particles to such a degree that the organels within the cell seemed to be distorted and pushed up against the cell wall. Dr. Johnson, therefore, suggested that the pathogenesis in these situations is cell death by internal crowding which alters cell metabolism, rather than by reactions usually associated with virus infections or hyperimmunity.

Aleutian mink virus presents a formidable challenge to work with, and yet, as Dr. Karstad stated, there are few viruses which are more tantalizing as models to investigate various aspects of pathogenesis. Aleutian mink virus produces a disease involving the reticuloendothelial system with the production of enormous quantities of gamma globulin; it appears to be a collagen disease; and there is mounting evidence that an important part of the pathogenesis is a hypersensitivity or an autoimmune phenomenon; and the expression of the disease has a genetic component.

Initially, the disease in mink was noted only in the double recessive Aleutian mink. For this reason there may be some confusion as to the role of the double recessive genetic trait and the role of the virus itself. Briefly, the genetic syndrome unrelated to the virus resembles that found in other animals and in humans (the Chidiak-Higashi syndrome) consisting of abnormal pigmentation, photophobia, increased light reflex, a striking increase of normal granular material in leukocytes, abnormal lipid metabolism and a general increased susceptibility to infections. In Aleutian mink the abnormal pigmentation results in a beautiful bluish coat which is valuable and highly sought after.

The Aleutian mink virus itself is capable of producing pathology in all types of mink, either wild or bred in colonies. The virus, however, is far more pathogenic for Aleutian mink with the double recessive gene.

Dr. Karstad presented new evidence supporting the role of hypersensitivity in Aleutian mink disease. A single inoculation of endotoxin produced a Shwartzman-like phenomenon in infected mink, and erythrocytes of infected animals gave positive Coombs tests. He believes that the most useful working hypothesis for pathogenesis of Aleutian mink disease involves a primary immune tolerance followed by waning of the tolerant state.

Because of the difficulties in working with Aleutian mink virus, progress has been at the characteristic pace of slow viruses. The agent has not been adapted to other hosts so that studies have to be conducted in mink, an expensive and unpleasant animal to work with. No tissue culture system is known which supports virus growth. Neither have conventional attempts to measure antibody been successful, and to date no antibody of any sort has been demonstrated to the Aleutian mink virus. Because of this and the fact that the organism is unusually resistant to heat and the effect of both DNAse and RNAse and other proteolytic enzymes, we might be well advised to refer to it as an agent rather than a virus, until it can be better characterized.

The studies of visna virus in sheep choroid plexus tissue culture by Dr. Thormar are impressive and truly the envy of other workers in the slow virus field. Visna, unlike other slow viruses, has been well defined. Animals suffering from the disease produce neutralizing antibody and there is a tissue culture system in which the virus can be propagated and causes cytopathic effects. In this sense visna is the only proved virus in the group, and it would be, perhaps, more proper to refer to the other infectious particles as "agents" as mentioned above with Aleutian mink disease. Visna virus in sheep is perhaps the most suitable animal model for the study of demyelinization although Waksman and Adams (1962) have commented that the demyelinization in visna differs to some extent from that of multiple sclerosis, allergic encephalitis and postinfectious encephalitis.

A most intriguing situation exists in the relationship between visna and maedi viruses, both of which have been studied in Iceland. The virus of visna and maedi are closely related serologically and in physical and cultural characteristics. The visna virus, however, causes disease in the central nervous system involving progressive demyelinization and death, while maedi virus causes pulmonary adenomatosis with no central nervous system manifestations.

In both diseases the pathology progresses in the presence of high titers of neutralizing antibody. Dr. Thormar showed that visna penetrates the cell more rapidly than it can be neutralized. He, therefore, suggested that visna virus could be carried in a protected state by blood elements and released near cells which it could infect before being neutralized. It, is also possible that either the virus is never in contact with antibody and spreads directly from cell to cell in the CNS or that the antibody itself is not competent, or that the antibody-virus complex is, itself, pathogenic.

Using his tissue culture technique Dr. THORMAR showed that virus replication is dependent on a transient increase in cellular DNA from 2–8 hours after inoculation although infectious virus does not appear for 15–20 hours.

Virus replication was completely suppressed by BUDR for up to 8 hours following inoculation, but addition of this transport DNA antagonist had no effect on virus multiplication if given after 8 hours. The suggestion is that an early alteration in the host cell was necessary in order for the infectious particle to develop. It is probable that a genetic-metabolic alteration occurred which apparently was preventable but not reversible. The phenomenon of an early change in the cell's metabolism which subsequently permits development of virus and attendant cell destruction is yet another fascinating possible mechanism of the pathogenesis for slow viruses.

Dr. HOTCHIN's provocative talk illustrated the problems of chronic infections and provided an immunological approach to the understanding of chronic virus diseases. Using the LCM virus, Dr. HOTCHIN has conducted a series of experiments on primary immune tolerance in mice. Recently he observed a phenomenon in mice with primary immune tolerance to LCM which he refers to as late disease, in which the animals have no overt signs of infections but age and die several months before uninfected mice. Development of late disease is dependent upon the strain of mouse and the route of inoculation. It is not yet clear whether late disease was caused by the LCM virus or by response to another factor, either infectious or toxic, in these unusual mice. Dr. HOTCHIN postulated that the development of late disease is related to the waning of tolerance or perhaps the actual development of hyperimmunity and suggested a similar mechanism in the pathogenesis of slow virus diseases. This would explain the long interval between infection and the development of clinical illness.

It will be recalled that earlier in the day Dr. JOHNSON pointed out another mechanism by which virus could remain in the host for long periods in the absence of symptoms. In JOHNSON's system viruses such as rabies were able to accumulate within cells while producing very little overt pathology. He postulated that after a certain point the accumulation of virus within the cell is so great that it alters cell metabolism and causes death. The accumulation is slow and the number of cells which must be destroyed is enormous before the animal shows clinical evidence of disease. His theory of the pathogenesis of slow viruses does not depend in any way upon the immune response.

Dr. THORMAR's theory of host cell-virus balance does not depend on the immune response to explain the pathogenesis in the systems which he studies. Using tissue culture models he postulated that the viruses of maedi and visna infected the mesenchymal tissue of the lung or CNS respectively. In explants he showed that the relationship between the cells and the virus stabilized and the culture was not completely destroyed. He was able to manipulate the degree of destruction of cells by changing the serum concentration of his media. This, he suggested, could be analogous to the situation *in vivo* and would explain how the virus could be present but in homeostasis for long periods of time and only become manifest when adverse environmental conditions developed.

It is probable that, as we learn more about viruses which cause chronic disease, we will find that the immunologic component in pathogenesis differs from disease to disease. Theoretically, three situations are possible. First, pathology can be the result of hypoactivity of the immune mechanism. Multifocal leukoencephalopathy, a progressive fatal disease of the central nervous system, occurs only in individuals with leukemia or other diseases of the reticuloendothelial system and possibly represents the action of a virus which the host can no longer maintain in check. Virus-like particles have been observed in the brains of people who died of multifocal leukoencephalopathy by electron microscopy (zu RHEIN and CHOU, 1965). Another interesting example of the effect of a virus in a hypoimmune host is measles infection in children with leukemia where in many instances the rash does not develop and instead there is a progressive giant cell pneumonia which is usually fatal.

A second possibility in the pathogenesis of chronic infections is one which is not dependent on the immune mechanism and can occur in the presence of a normal immune response. An instance of this would be Dr. JOHNSON's suggestion about rabies. Also, it would be possible that virus not multiplying in central nervous system tissue causes central nervous system degeneration by suppression or stimulation of a particular metabolite or hormone or even the abnormal consumption of a metabolite. Nerve cells are extremely vulnerable since they cannot replicate and have no storage capacity, particularly for oxidative metabolism.

The third possibility is that of prolonged infection leading to a state of hypersensitivity against the virus, as Dr. HOTCHIN suggested in late disease with LCM, or against a nonspecific or shared antigen as has been suggested in multiple sclerosis and rheumatoid arthritis. There are some interesting data (PATTISON, 1966) concerning scrapie which suggest a possible hyperimmune state. In goats if normal brain material was inoculated intraperitoneally and subsequently scrapie brain material was given, the incubation period was considerably reduced. Also, when scrapie virus was inoculated subcutaneously, those animals which had a local reaction at the site of injection developed symptoms several months sooner than those animals in which a local reaction was not observed.

Dr. GIBBS presented recent findings which indicate that kuru, a chronic fatal infection of man, is transmissible to chimpanzees. The data of course are preliminary, but among 30 chimpanzees inoculated with human brain material from patients who died of various causes, only those chimpanzees which received material from kuru patients have become ill. The symptoms resembled kuru and appeared from 18 to 25 months after inoculation. Preliminary neuropathological examination revealed lesions similar to those observed in kuru. It is unlikely that the reaction was an allergic encephalitis since the chimpanzees received only one dose of inoculum and the symptoms did not appear for 18 months. Further, the pathology did not resemble allergic encephalitis. A remote possibility is that the inoculum was contaminated with scrapie virus. Pathologically the lesions in kuru are virtually indistinguishable from those of scrapie. Since no antibody system has been developed for either kuru or scrapie, it may be some time before the relationship between these diseases is worked out and conclusive proof obtained that the lesions seen in chimpanzees were not caused by the scrapie virus as a laboratory contaminant. Another remote possibility, *in view* of the fact that filtered material has not yet produced symptoms, is that a parasitic or bacterial agent endemic in New Guinea is responsible for these lesions in chimpanzees.

The work which Dr. GIBBS presented concerning scrapie virus underscores the exciting and yet frustrating and bewildering position in which we find ourselves in the field of slow viruses. Initially, scrapie was thought to be a genetic disease. With the accumulation of evidence, it is now difficult to deny that this disease is caused by a transmissible agent, probably viral, with a strong genetic component. The impression one gets from the literature and from discussions with other workers is that the agent is pathogenic for many if not all species tested, although some animals must be observed for a very long time before symptoms develop.

To date no system has been developed to detect antibody to the scrapie virus. It may be that we are dealing with a naked RNA particle or other poorly antigenic substance. We may also have a situation analogous to that with the LDH virus of mice in which antibody cannot be detected by routine methods because it is bound in an unusual way to the virus. Recent advances in cancer research open new areas for speculation concerning the possibilities of helper viruses and subviral particles.

The scrapie agent invades the reticuloendothelial system several weeks or months before it appears in the central nervous system. The pathology observed, however, is almost entirely confined to the central nervous system. The agent is difficult to isolate from blood. By routine tests it has not been demonstrated to produce interferon and has not been visualized by electron microscopy. The infectious particle is incredibly resistant to inactivation by heat, UV light, and even formalin. Attempts to document the size of the infectious particle have yielded conflicting results. When studied by gradocol filtration the agent is in the range of 20 mμ, and cesium-chloride density gradient centrifugation indicated that it is a nucleoprotein free of lipids. There are, however, reports that the infectious particle is dialyzable. Most recently ALPER (1966) calculated the "target size" of scrapie from radiation inactivation data and suggested that the infectious particle is about five mμ in diameter. This would mean that it is too small to contain nucleic acid.

Clearly a great deal of work remains to be done with this agent and the others in the slow virus group. Progress will not be fast since each experiment takes months or years, and with the exception of visna there are still no tissue culture systems or antibody systems with which to study. Many of the experiments already reported must be repeated since the findings of different groups are at variance with each other and in several instances are totally unexplainable within our present concept of infectious agents.

I would like to take the liberty to conclude by quoting a poem which I believe expresses our present position. These are the last six lines of a sonnet by Keats entitled "On First Looking into Chapman's Homer", in which the poet describes the discovery of the Pacific and the emotion felt by the explorers.

> "... Then felt I like some watcher of the skies
> When a new planet swims into his ken;
> Or like stout Cortez when with eagle eyes
> He stared at the Pacific — and all his men
> Looked at each other with a wild surmise —
> Silent, upon a peak in Darien."

While this sonnet expresses the excitement we all feel at the possibility that we are launching into a new area in the understanding of infectious disease, it is most appropriate to point out that Mr. Keats had not succeeded in getting his facts straight. After all, it was not Cortez but Balboa who discovered the Pacific.

References

Alper, T., D. A. Haig, and M. C. Clarke: The exceptionally small size of the scrapie agent. Biochem. biophys. Res. Commun. **22**, 278—283 (1966).

Brody, J.A., W. J. Hadlow, J. Hotchin, R. T. Johnson, H. Koprowski, and L. T. Kurland: Soviet search for viruses that cause chronic neurologic diseases in the U.S.S.R. Science **147**, 1114—1116 (1965).

Gajdusek, D. C.: Kuru in New Guinea and the origin of the NINDB study of slow, latent, and temperate virus infections of the nervous system of man. In: Slow, Latent, and Temperate Virus Infections, NINDB Monograph No. 2, PHS Publication No. 1378 (1965).

Pattison, I. H.: Experiments with scrapie with special reference to the nature of the agent and the pathology of the disease. In: Slow, Latent, and Temperate Virus Infections, NINDB Monograph No. 2, PHS Publication No. 1387 (1966).

Reed, D., C. Plato, T. Elizan, and L. T. Kurland: The amyotrophic lateral sclerosis/parkinsonism-dementia complex: A ten-year follow-up on Guam. Part I. Epidemiologic studies. Amer. J. Epidem. **83**, 54—73 (1966).

Waksman, B. H., and R. D. Adams: Infectious leukoencephalitis. J. Neuropath. exp. Neurol. **21**, 491—518 (1962).

Zlotnik, I.: Observations on the experimental transmission of scrapie of various origins to laboratory animals. In: Slow, Latent, and Temperate Virus Infections, NINDB Monograph No. 2, PHS Publication. No. 1378 (1965).

Zu Rhein, G. M., and S. M. Chou: Particles resembling papova viruses in human cerebral demyelinating disease. Science **148**, 1477—1479 (1965).

Subject Index

The numbers printed in *italics* refer to illustrations.
Letter "T" after the page numbers points to catch words, mentioned in a table.

Offsetdruck: Julius Beltz, Weinheim/Bergstr.

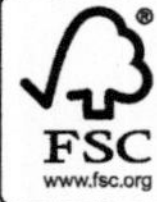

MIX
Papier aus verantwortungsvollen Quellen
Paper from responsible sources
FSC® C105338

If you have any concerns about our products,
you can contact us on
ProductSafety@springernature.com

In case Publisher is established outside the EU,
the EU authorized representative is:
Springer Nature Customer Service Center GmbH
Europaplatz 3, 69115 Heidelberg, Germany

Printed by Libri Plureos GmbH
in Hamburg, Germany